MAYBE BABY

Matthew M. F. Miller

An Infertile Love Story

Health Communications, Inc.
Deerfield Beach, Florida

www.hcibooks.com

Library of Congress Cataloging-in-Publication Data

Miller, Matthew M. F.
  Maybe baby / Matthew M. F. Miller.
    p. cm.
  ISBN-13: 978-0-7573-0748-5 (trade paper)
  ISBN-10: 0-7573-0748-5 (trade paper)
  1. Miller, Matthew M. F. 2. Childlessness—United States—Psychological
aspects. 3. Infertility—United States—Psychological aspects. I. Title.
  HQ536.M53 2008
  306.87—dc22

                                                                    2008022744

Publisher: Health Communications, Inc.
          3201 S.W. 15th Street
          Deerfield Beach, FL 33442-8190

Cover images by Orion Johnson
Cover design by Andrea Perrine Brower
Interior design by Dawn Von Strolley Grove
Formatting by Lawna Patterson Oldfield

This book is dedicated to my beautiful and intelligent wife, Constance, without whom this story would have never been told. I mean, I can't *not* get pregnant by myself, now can I? In other words, thank you for being mine. Your love is limitless.

"Familiarity breeds contempt—and children."

—**Mark Twain**, author

"Football (soccer) is a fertility festival. Eleven sperm trying to get into the egg. I feel sorry for the goalkeeper."

—**Björk**, Icelandic singer-songwriter

"The difficulty of IVF or of any fertility issues is the hope and the shattered hope, the dream that it might happen this time and then it doesn't happen."

—**Brooke Shields**, actress

Contents

• •

Contents

Introduction

· ·

Welcome to Planet Infertility:
Six Million Strong . . . and Growing

We live in a world of circles; a world of hereditary life cycles, seasons, and orbits; of culs-de-sac and lint-covered Butter Rum Lifesavers circa who-knows-when rescued from the pocket of an overcoat you thought you'd donated to the Salvation Army years ago. Like everything cyclical, what once reeked of cliché becomes new again upon finding yourself right back where you started, and that coat you should have tossed out is now at the pinnacle of style. Even the aged Lifesavers, albeit inexplicably white in color, are still capable of saving your life at the most inopportune of garlic-breath moments.

Never is this circle more pronounced than in the reproductive arena. It's a racetrack upon which the dreams, genes, and genitalia of two people unite to create a next generation hybrid who will carry on the physical traits and legacies of said people once the curtain has closed on their limited earthbound engagements. Circles give everyone and everything a chance to renew what otherwise would simply cease to exist.

My name is Matthew Miller, I'm twenty-nine years old, and I am an infertile man. My sperm counts fluctuate by tens of millions of swimmers, and for whatever reason, they never seem to be available in bulk when it matters most. And like every other "infertile" who has come before me and every "infertile" who will battle hence, I live life on a straight line.

My wife, Constance, and I have been trying to conceive our first child for more than two years. During that time, we have moved from simple intercourse to semen analyses, from Clomid to insemination, from simple procreation science to the artifice of in vitro fertilization without so much as a layover. We always told ourselves that we wouldn't be the people who'd take it this far—that if, for some reason, we couldn't get pregnant we'd adopt—but once you consent to living life on a straight line there is nowhere to get off until you arrive at the end.

Every month, every fresh cycle, and every new treatment feels like it could finally terminate the constant view of rocky terrain ahead, of the never-ending mountain that kicks your ass day after day. Infertility treatment is a carrot-on-a-stick with tight brown curls and a paisley onesie that tempts you to run harder and faster while always dangling the coveted two-line pregnancy test just out of reach. Constance and I keep chugging along with the expectation that one day we will open our eyes to an effortless downhill track, a clear view of the sun, and nothing but momentum and forgiveness at our backs. So far, the only things at my back are a few more errant hairs in need of waxing.

I continue to get older, more tired, and more hopeful that, if there's not a child ahead, at least there's a relaxing day spa employing the world's strongest masseuse buried somewhere in this impenetrable cliff. So far, no such luck.

As Iowa's Little Hawkeye Math Champion in eighth grade, it was my responsibility to spread the numerical gospel that the shortest path between any two points is a straight line. Today, sixteen years removed from my coronation, I'm afraid if that basic principle holds true, then I don't know what my destination is. Unless my life turns, there will be nothing for me to leave behind in this world other than my work and the love I've given to my family. Like any challenge, however, it has made me the man I am today—a loving husband, a struggling writer, and proud brother, son, and uncle—and I like being me. Perhaps a straight line won't be the fastest way to get to our baby, but I believe we will get there regardless because I can't help but imagine what I would be, what I could be, once my line is allowed to bend into a circle.

This book is about our struggle with infertility, but more

than that, it's about the love, laughter, and hope that two people in love share when they trust and respect each other enough to replicate. It's the story of two normal people in love trying to overcome one more challenge in a world chockfull of challenges.

And unlike our reproductive efforts, it's just that simple.

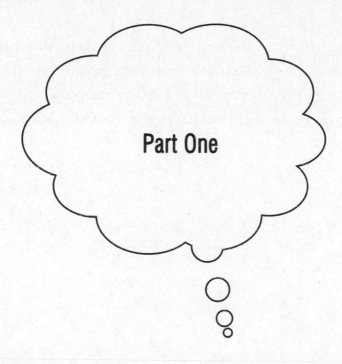

Part One

First Comes Love, Then Comes
Marriage, Then Comes . . .

Chapter 1

· ·

Meth Houses, Red Delicious Apples, and Infertile People

Inside the peeling, mustard-yellow house of my youth, there remained an outside possibility that our firstborn child would be conceived in my childhood bedroom, on my parents' hand-me-down bed, twenty-nine years following my creation under the same modest roof on the same lumpy mattress. I was not born in my hometown of Peru, Iowa, because there is no hospital to serve its one hundred and twenty residents born to farming, building, and low-paying desk jobs. I was not born in nearby Winterset, birthplace of John Wayne and *The Bridges of Madison County*, home of my eventual high school, because the only hospital in our area code was not stocked or staffed with sufficient baby-fetching apparatus.

Even *in utero* I was destined for the city, and Des Moines was my parents' only viable metropolis without crossing state lines. During a pre-Christmas snowstorm, my pregnant mom sat passenger while my father drove forty-five minutes to Methodist Hospital where she gave birth to a nearly ten-pound bald monster child who would go on to become a nearly five-hundred-pound monster child by the age of sixteen before settling into life as a slim, healthy, bald twenty-nine-year-old writer.

My children will never know small-town life, will never know what it's like to live where cows and graves outnumber the citizens of their hometown. They will never know my Peru childhood, the hours eating in front of the television, without a library or shopping mall within twenty miles, the endless filling of my mouth with junk foods and leftovers to fill the unstructured hours that ticked by completely unnoticed.

But after seventeen months of unsuccessfully trying to conceive, I would have given anything to give my children a future, to give Hugo or Iris life, even in a place where I found none.

It was Thanksgiving night, my belly full of Midwest-style salads that always contained Jell-O but never a vegetable, and I lay on my back dabbing the sweat off my forehead with a pair of hastily discarded boxer shorts. Plowing the itchy foam blanket into a wall between Constance and me in order to deflect the heat of her sleep-induced steam, I sat up in bed and reached for my red-framed Dolce & Gabbana glasses on the bedside table. It must have been eighty degrees in the airless room, and I needed to clear the dollhouse and princess vanity from the end of the bed in order to gain access to the grate, close the vents, and diffuse the heat generated from our active bodies and the overactive furnace. Dad was a furnace and air man, and the one thousand square feet we called home shifted between extremes of heat and cold, depending on the season, was proof of his mastery of the ductile arts.

Situated in the northwest corner of the house, my old bedroom, located on the opposite side of the world when compared to our minimalist Chicago bedroom, was always the warmest in the winter and the coldest in the summer of any of the house's five rooms. Before I took up residence, my sisters had shared those bright yellow walls for sixteen years, arguing over the division of territory and where it was appropriate for the Bon Jovi posters to end and the Ozzy Osborne posters to begin.

Once Angie got married and April moved to Des Moines to share an apartment with her boyfriend in a house otherwise occupied by Bosnian refugees—a living arrangement that had my mother praying for her safety at the top of each hour—the coveted den of inequity was mine.

As a right of property passage, we all must have learned to pull the grate out of the floor and manually push the vents closed one by one after sex to avoid postcoital heat exhaustion. Peru (pronounced "pee-roo") is a formulaic small town with gutted buildings and a post office that's open only twelve hours each week. One stop sign stands in the center of town, positioned less than ten yards from my old bedroom window. It is less a traffic mandate for the tractors and Ford trucks that choose to ignore its presence than it is a warning to residents.

My old window has remained uncovered since the day I folded and packed my Philadelphia Eagles blanket that had served as a makeshift curtain across the single-pane window. It had hung from a row of red thumbtacks bolted to the fluorescent wall. The blanket since has become a favorite chew toy of our dogs, Hazel and Marcy, back in Chicago, and its threadbare fibers would no longer block much of the harsh street lamp that was burning through the west-facing glass.

Diagonally across the street from Peru's stop sign resides the town's solitary monument—mahogany-stained two-by-fours nailed together in the shape of an oversize water well. A flowerbed stands in place of a brick water shaft. No liquid can be retrieved, not from the fake monument and not from the barren silt-and-limestone creek across the road.

A four-inch, red-painted apple is branded into the top slats, followed by the ash-stained announcement:

WELCOME TO PERU, IOWA
HOME OF THE RED DELICIOUS APPLE
1887–1987

Peru's crowning achievement, the stump of the first red delicious apple tree, is located somewhere outside of town and battles for position with a fencepost at the top of a ditch. Its memorial, however, resides on the front lawn of the former site of the town's most notorious meth house, which burned to the ground in 2004. Mom says the flames that night made our house glow and that she felt like a lightning bug trapped in a jar full of burning leaves.

As I stood in the center of the window in a room with no clock, I could tell it was somewhere around eleven o'clock, more due to the muffled snippets of Leno than the position of the moon. Dad had always had been a Letterman guy until he visited Constance and me when we lived in Los Angeles and attended a *Tonight Show* taping. Since then, his allegiances to late-night television had been forever altered.

My thighs were burning from having sex on a worn-out mattress, a relic that hadn't offered support since the summer the Iran Contra Scandal preempted *All My Children*. I raised my left foot into my right hand behind me and stretched, imagining that I was gearing up for a ten-mile run, alternating back and forth until the compact knots in my calves loosened, leaving behind only a mild sting.

Constance wouldn't be ovulating for another five days, but having intercourse at this point was a safeguard and a sanity check. One more go for good measure.

One more go in the land of fertile farms and teenagers.

Most families I knew had at least one child that got pregnant in high school or at least before marriage, and mine was no exception. April got pregnant about a year after graduating and immediately became my hero for not getting married for another ten months following my niece's birth. April was controversial and cool and, in my eyes, lived at the apex of all things edgy.

As a kid I was afraid of sex. I was a revoltingly obese, 476 pounds at the peak of my high-school days, and in order to avoid the humiliation of disrobing in front of a perfect young woman and the possibility of unwanted fat descendants, I shunned full-on sex—all forms that required removal of undergarments and T-shirts—until I was no longer fat. Weight wasn't the only deterrent; it took only two knocked-up classmates to ruin it for Winterset Senior High's Class of 1997. When the girls got pregnant, I held, with religious fervor, a belief that I would end up a teenage father the first time I had sex. Which is why it probably seemed to Constance that my constant advances and arousals were an attempt to make up for bygone juvenilia. Especially on that day, in my childhood bedroom, where prior to loving her, I had never engaged in full-on sex.

My arousal on Thanksgiving Day was of culinary lineage. The stuffing had been a monumental disappointment, a watery, crunchy imposter, and disappointing food always made sex more urgent for me. I am a pleasure addict—food, sex, music—and if one avenue disappoints, it only serves to increase my needs and expectations for the others. Our sex had remained passionate five years into marriage, even now that it had a mission and a purpose that failed us time after time. Lousy stuffing only made the kisses warmer, gave the innocent nibbles on fragrant skin a bit more bite.

We were finally, after years of safety and prevention, having sex for the sake of sex's ultimate utility. Little had changed, however, except for the sixteen days over the course of sixteen months that began with bleeding and ended with disappointment.

Sex only seemed different now, in my mind, while standing in front of the window.

As if reading Braille I couldn't decipher, I rubbed my fingers across the scattershot holes where tacks once affixed Andre Agassi, Tori Amos, Monica Seles, and Michael Stipe to my walls. Holes that now were the only decorations left. Void of a frame, the mattress was pushed into the corner. Above it, three rows of shelves my dad had carved, sanded, and stained to house my music collection now housed every Disney movie and Shirley Temple videotape in existence. At the foot of the bed and to the left of the non-existent headboard were graveyards of abused, misfit toys my five nieces and nephews had long since discarded in favor of more age-appropriate, technologically savvy fare.

Sex never made sense in this room back when it was just for recreation, a shared wall with my parents' bedroom—an insufficient buffer for something so cliché. But the more we departed from the textbook definition of reproduction, the more this mishmash of past and present was as logical of a place as any to make our future Miller. Perhaps a manhandled Hulk Hogan and a butchered-until-butch Strawberry Shortcake would be the good luck tokens we needed.

"Maybe we should get drunk before we do it tonight," I'd said earlier that day as I ran my fingers through Constance's brown curls in the basement of the Peru United Methodist Church. Once Grandma J's house could no longer accommodate the expanding generations of our family, we'd moved all familial celebrations to the dank underbelly of the town's only house of worship, which always smelled like sweaty sneakers and balsa wood. "I mean, it's worked so well for so long for so many young people in this neck of the woods. Why not us?"

"Hey, you never know," Constance had said, driving her stuffing around a paper plate with a plastic fork until it was no longer touching any of her other lunch items. "Nothing like cheap vodka to start your baby out on the right foot." We both laughed, and I lowered my mouth to meet the skin on the back of her neck, above the first notch of her spine, with a kiss that I knew would make my intentions clear.

But now, as I continued to stare into the rural night, sex was no longer on my mind. Three inches of snow were stacked like a load of whites on top of the discarded washer and dryer sitting in the bed of Dad's freight trailer parked in the side yard. My eyes darted back and forth between the stop sign, the broken-down laundry apparatus, and the red delicious apple sign as I listened to the deepening breaths of Constance's sleep mixed with occasional outbursts from Leno's studio audience.

I surveyed the visual buffet before me—stop sign, trailer, red delicious apple, burned bits of the meth house—and I tried to turn it all into something more than the nothing it always represented. Something that could make sense out of why we couldn't conceive and why everyone around us could.

I wanted to take the meth ashes, the traffic warnings, and the truth of a sterile town and turn them into something that would make me feel like a father.

Someone should clear away the debris from the meth house, I thought. *It's been three years.*

Chapter 2

. . . .

Pottery Barn, Wendy Spizziri, and Evil Catalogs

Once upon a time, on the top story of a two-flat apartment on the north side of Chicago, a tattered, unsolicited catalog arrived in the mailbox of Matthew and Constance Miller. And with it came an undefined, yuppie-prescribed voodoo that, within a few flips of its pages, unleashed a punishing kaleidoscope of pinks, blues, greens, and yellows that struck us, the aforementioned Millers, immediately infertile.

David and Alison Archibald we were not, but a quick inspection of the label allowed us to conclude that indeed we were the "or current residents" also listed as possible recipients of such junk mail. On the cover were two babies, one girl and one boy, both white, both bitten and scarred by the cruel postal machine, and both wrapped in terrycloth animal towels with hoods, one in the shape of a frog and the other a giraffe.

"I swear, Pottery Barn would send these catalogs to my barren grandmother for the chance to kill just one more tree," I said, tossing the catalog onto the sofa next to Constance. Her eyes were locked into the Food Network's Saturday morning lineup, never once shifting away from pots and pans to meet my eyes or those of the children on the front of the publication.

Ina Garten's over-cheesed polenta—a corn-based lava flowing out of the saucepan and into a buttered baking dish—pushed my wife's mind into a prison of pernicious food pornography. Words could not penetrate the reinforced walls of her culinary jail.

"What?" she asked, staring straight ahead at the televised tractor beam that was pulling her deeper into a cooking world where my words were foreign obscenities and heavy whipping cream was god.

"You're not listening to me," I said, rapping my knuckles on my head, knocking my scalp. "Hello, McFly!"

"Yes, I am," she said. "You said something about Pottery Barn and your grandma's trees."

"No, that's not what I said at all. You are impossible while the TV is on."

Constance broke her gaze as my idealized disappointment rang true. Lifting the remote, she jabbed it at the screen until the sound disappeared and only Ina's cheese-covered spatula continued to spread the good word of great French cuisine.

"I'm sorry, Matty," she said. "What did you say?"

"Nothing, never mind," I said, plopping down on the opposite end of the oversize purple sofa, the cushions swallowing me

until I was perfectly molded into its body. "Just watch Ina. It's
no big deal. I'll sit here and talk to myself about really important things while you enjoy your program."

"You're a poop," she laughed.

Constance picked up the magazine and threw the tattered
tots and their overpriced adornments at my torso, only her
poor aim sent it on a collision course with the side of my head.
Children of the rich and privileged with names like Jack and
Hannah, all dressed in impossible sweaters and dresses and
tights more perfect than I had ever owned. And yet they were
the youngest humans I had ever resented because they were
everything I secretly wanted.

"Ewww, get it off me!" I yelled, picking up the corners of
the catalog as if every child between the staples had used it as
a makeshift diaper.

"You wanna look at it with me?" she asked.

Two years previous, we had moved from Los Angeles to
Chicago, from the ocean and mountains of excess to expansive
flatness and frugality, from eighteen thousand dollars in credit
card debt to the realization that we were shopping junkies
always in search of the next good fix. Our new friend, Krista
Thomas, a six-foot tall, fast-talking Chicago native who knew
how to hold her tequila and dance the two-step, had gone to

college with a burgeoning financial consultant, and after she and Constance talked about the ills of our finances, she said we just had to meet Wendy.

"She'll change your life," she'd told us. "She really knows her shit."

Following one session with Wendy Spizirri, we were left with no choices and no option but to believe that every delivery order of pad thai we made might taste sweet and nutty, but not as sweet and nutty as a zero balance on all of our cards. Wendy's sincere, innocent blue eyes and mass of crisp brown curls attached to her skull like a war helmet were to us like a rescued puppy looking for a loving, debt-free home. A home where kibble was plentiful and its purchase wasn't attached to an eighteen-percent interest rate. Wendy was our doe-eyed dog, and it was our responsibility to provide her a fiscally accountable home.

In our first act of adulthood, we bought life insurance, enough to supplement the loss of our incomes for three years in the case of death, but we held off investing in a money market account until our debt was paid off.

"Let's feed the monster before we cook our own ramen noodles," I'd said, pleased with my clever analogy in the face of numbers and planning that were dripping, unused, off the sides of my creative palette.

"I don't get it," Constance had said. "What do you mean by that?"

Quizzical stares were abundant in our home. Constance was an absolute pragmatist; I was an abstract painter, and my picture was always replete with flourishes and splatters. Hers might as well have been a window.

"I just mean, we should kill the debt before we invest," I'd explained.

"Are you guys planning on having children?" Wendy had asked, as she flipped through the fill-in-the-blank book that quickly had become a dossier on our gluttony, the "before" pictures replete with wrinkles and love handles. "Because a money market account will be great when the little one arrives to help cover lost salaries and the added expenses. Are you planning a family?"

"We are someday," Constance had said. "I've been accruing leave at work, and as soon as I have three months of sick time and our credit cards are paid off, we're going to start trying. Both of those things are really important to us."

"But that's still a ways off," I'd added. "We've got a lot of debt and not much sick time. And that hungry monster to feed." Constance rolled her eyes and shook her head as if to dismiss my embarrassing repeat attempt to make the monster/ramen-noodle analogy succeed.

Wendy instructed Constance and me each to grab a shovel and begin digging ourselves out of the chic Pottery Barn grave we had been throwing dirt on top of for more than three years. Cans of tuna fish for lunches, boxed soups for dinner, basic cable for entertainment, running fifteen hundred miles in my shoes before buying a new pair: each slash of the budget brought us closer to ground level and to those inevitable next steps. First comes marriage, then comes life insurance, then comes baby in an affordable baby carriage.

"How did it get this bad?" I'd asked, flipping through the credit card statements spread out in front of us. Evidence proved to Wendy that we, when left to our own devices, were incapable of moderation. "There's no way we can have a kid until this is taken care of. It would be unconscionable to bring a child into this world with our finances like this."

"Yeah, it'll be a while before we can start thinking about that," Constance had said. "Plus, I want to get a little more physically prepared." Constance had been trying to lose ten to twenty pounds since I had known her, always pulling clothes against her stomach and frowning into the mirror, but I had always thought her body was a perfect Victorian painting.

Sitting with Wendy, I stared at eighteen thousand dollars spread across six credit card statements and one peasant-style dining room table. It was the debt equivalent of a blood splatter analysis in the pages of a mass-market crime thriller. I could have easily poured over every detail of this creditors' novella in an attempt to recreate our crime, but it was unnecessary to critique each drop of blood to ascertain the truth. Constance and I were addicted to style.

Specifically, a blend of modern and Shaker.

Truth was threaded through every inch of the six-hundred-dollar Oriental rug we couldn't afford to buy out-of-pocket and instead put on the MasterCard. Truth was sixteen sticks of bamboo, sixteen costly focal points jutting up from the center of a sleek, curvy coffee table for which a twenty-something budget didn't allow. Truth was woven into the fabric of the triple-digit chenille throw and thousand-dollar designer bedding that threw our income-to-lifestyle ratio into an inequitable tailspin.

Unlike many women of her generation, Constance never wanted to be Carrie Bradshaw. She only wanted to sleep each night on the same floral-print Calvin Klein bedding featured prominently in her staged Manhattan flat. Unfortunately for her, when we began our descent into debt in 2001, I was not a functional, profiteering writer like the fictional Ms. Bradshaw. In fact, my craft had shifted from words to the artless construction of end-cap toilet paper mountains at a suburban Minneapolis Target. Supporting my new wife during her graduate work at the University of Minnesota was a labor bred partially of love and partially of a red-and-khaki-clothed depression.

Two nights and one day a week, I would drive from the Minnetonka Super Target to the Mall of America, swap my red polo shirt for a black T-shirt, and lodge myself in the stuffed stockroom at Pottery Barn. A Tetris obsession that had me skipping Principles of Reasoning during my first year at the University of Iowa served me well as I spent countless four-hour shifts shuffling stock to make room for three more Malabar chairs in a world already congested by Malabar chairs.

My steep employee discounts lured Constance and me into thinking that percentages off added up to something we should take advantage of in lieu of bona fide cash to pay the remaining percentages. Nesting newlyweds, we felt choked by the out-of-style, hand-me-down bookcases and the ancient oak-boxed television, a two-hundred-pound behemoth on a swivel. The screen emitted a thin rainbow that ran through the center of the screen but with no pot of gold or even decent reception for *Buffy the Vampire Slayer* on the other side. Sleeping on the floor on a mattress and box springs with no bed frame, covered by Constance's flowery teenaged bedding, made us feel suffocated by shabbiness. Cooking without a Kitchen-Aid mixer and anodized skillets could never allow me to create the gourmet foods whipped up by stars of the Food Network. DKNY sweaters framed my broad shoulders and elongated torso better than frumpy mass-market apparel designed for frumpy, mass-market people. We both had a desire to be something, to be those people in catalogs, and in order to achieve yuppie nirvana, we bought the overpriced goods that all successful twenty-somethings in the catalogs owned.

Two years later, our sieve leaked thousands more in moving expenses en route to Los Angeles. Constance took a job with the U.S. Air Force's space program for one year, sidestepping her women's policy dreams to monitor billions in defense spending, while I worked toward my Masters in Professional Writing at the University of Southern California. Keeping up with the LA lifestyle, the exorbitant rents, and six-dollar gallons of milk pushed me, a nonswimmer, further beneath the flood. Constance and I wanted out—out of our jobs, out of our celebrity-focused surroundings, and out of our debt that was drowning us. So we moved to Chicago, drove our PT Cruiser through Arizona, New Mexico, Texas, Oklahoma, Kansas, Iowa, and Illinois, in search of a fresh start.

So when Constance cracked the pages of the Pottery Barn Kids catalog that day, it was like seeing an alcoholic sniff the dregs of an empty wine glass. I slid across the sofa until my left leg bonded to her right. I draped my arm around her back, dipping my fingertips into the waistband of her drawstring pants, and kissed her forehead. One credit card with a four-thousand-dollar balance was all that remained, and talk of babies had been more frequent in the past few months. Yet I still doubted the robustness of our rehabilitation, whether or not we could dip our toes into the Pottery Barn pool again without diving in headfirst.

Children would happen for us in the near term, but not until Constance's work leave accrued to cover ninety days post-delivery in June. And not until the last dollar of debt was paid off. But the knowledge of almost enough time off and

almost no debt had become an embedded alarm clock emitting childlike screams in my ears—screams that would not
allow me to stop thinking about our own future children.
Which made the arrival of the catalog even scarier for two
out-of-control spenders within sniffing distance of both a finish line and a starting line.

"Wow, that's really awesome," I said, jabbing my finger at
the affluent nursery set only four pages into the catalog. Mint
green walls covered with stick-on birds migrating toward a
wall cling in the shape of a stoic oak tree decorated the layout.
Cream bedding with green accents and the most charming,
pretentious farm animal–backed quilt were spread between
the walls of a picturesque crib lined with a matching bumper.
It was as if Winnie-the-Pooh and friends had relocated to a
charming Iowa homestead following the razing of the hun-
dred-acre woods to make way for condos.

"Matty, that's perfect!" Constance backhanded my forearm
with excited aggression and thrust the magazine within an
inch of my nose. Since childhood, Constance had been labeled
a bull in a china shop by her mother, Susan, and now that she
was all mine, I had been anointed as her very own flesh-and-
blood Lennox outlet.

"I know," I said as I pushed the magazine back down onto
my lap. "It's really great."

"No, Matty, I don't think you understand," she said, pushing the page closer to my eyes until the slick paper scraped my

nose. "I'm really picky about stuff like this. I have never seen a nursery set I've even kind of liked. It's always so hokey and too gender specific. Manufacturers always stick girls in princess-themed rooms with nothing but pink.

"It's true," I said. "It's why I hate going to Victoria's Secret. It's like being trapped inside of a giant vagina. Or a vagina gift box."

"Matty, I'm serious. This is the first time I've ever found one I really like." Constance's volume evaporated from a full, ebullient Chicago alto to a whisper by the time she arrived at her final word. It was a trick that had come to signal the seriousness of an inquiry, be it a request for another pair of black shoes or more after-dinner dark chocolate. When her voice dissipated, I knew she was asking permission to make a request she knew I'd find unnecessary.

"Well, what do you want?" I asked.

"I don't know," she said, each word descending softer in volume and ascending higher in pitch until I had no choice but to offer the solution I knew she sought.

"Do you want to buy it?"

"Yes, but is that ridiculous? That's ridiculous isn't it?"

"Yeah, it kinda is," I said. "I mean, we don't have a kid and we haven't even started trying for one yet."

"I know, but we'll have one someday," Constance said. "And even if we can't have one for some reason, we'll adopt. It'll get used."

"Whatever you want to do. I mean, it is totally cool by me. We can keep it in storage until we need it."

"Are you serious?" she asked. "I know it's ridiculous, but I'm worried that if we don't get it now, when we do need one, I'll never find one I like and this will haunt me."

"That's a valid concern," I said, kissing her once again on the forehead and laughing. "I can't have my baby being haunted by nonbuyer's remorse. Why don't you go ahead and order it? I mean, we spend our money on worse things all the time. I think you should go for it."

Constance leapt from the sofa and grabbed the phone. "Matty, can you get my wallet? I'm gonna need the debit card." After fetching her wallet, I dropped down into the plank position and began doing my daily penance of two hundred and fifty push-ups, eight hundred stomach crunches, and five hundred butt-lifts. Ina Garten was gone, and Rachael Ray had taken her place, pounding garlic cloves with the flat end of a Füri knife with an aggression equal to my up-and-down thrusts, face to floor, as I listened to Constance's one-sided order.

"Oh, really? Wow, then I'm glad I called. And we didn't really want the bumper anyway."

Silence.

"Yes, we want the wall cling, the quilt, and the valance."

Silence.

"That's fine. How long will the cling be on back order?"

Silence.

"Perfect. I'd like to pay with a Visa." Digits flowed into the phone, the sixteen numbers of her debit card issued to the customer representative, a pay-for-it-now purchase that proved we were the kind of people who believed that buying on time would eventually steal our future.

"Oh, no, we're not pregnant," Constance said. "That's okay, it's sweet of you to offer congratulations. This is just the first nursery set I've ever liked and thought I should go ahead and get it because we'll have a baby soon."

Constance hung up the phone, placed the catalog and the receiver on the cushions of the sofa, and then crawled on her knees toward me, reenacting Michelle Pfeiffer's seductive cat crawl from *Batman Returns,* and rested her head on my stomach.

"Your belly is so firm," she said, running circles with her finger across my tense abdomen. "I'm so glad we found that bedding."

Chapter 3

. . . .

The First and Fourth Times I Knew I Wanted to Be a Father

I scribbled my name across the brown electronic pad for the third time and thanked the UPS man for his patience. Perfectionist tendencies plagued me, and the first two times I signed for the package, I created one sloping mountain followed by a downward spiking line that dribbled out of the signing window before my scrawl ever reached the middle. By the third go, the two flourishing *m*'s that designate my first and last names were the only legible letters.

"That'll be just fine," the deliveryman said as he yanked the pad out of my hands and darted down the front steps. He leapt like a skittish deer into his double-parked truck and drove away before I had a chance to request a fourth attempt.

"It's here," I yelled from the bottom of the twisting stairs leading up to our apartment. Skipping every other step, I sprinted so quickly to the top, leaping over two napping cats sprawled out on separate stairs, that Constance had yet to make it from the kitchen to the dining room to greet me. The box was heavier than I expected, which was a comfort. Thicker fibers and better-quality materials would keep our baby warm in a breezy old apartment that never heated above sixty-four degrees.

"I wanna open it," Constance yelled, shaking her fist, which held the red meat scissors rarely used to cut once-living creatures. She poked the splayed blades through the thick brown tape that sealed the lid.

"Don't stick it in too deep," I said. "You don't want to hurt it."

"That's what *she* said," Constance quipped.

"Don't be a pervert in front of our baby's bedding. You don't want it to get the right idea about us."

Once the tape was cleared, I pulled open the flaps, and then Constance reached in to grab the filler, slowly ruffling the magic curtain of crumpled paper topping the items hidden beneath. Finally we owned something for a child we had always wanted, but a child we never thought would come.

"Here we go," she said. "I can't believe we're really about to see this. Our first baby bedding."

"I love you," I said as I leaned over the box, her hand still quivering on the paper, and kissed her perfect lips. Parting them with my tongue, I was flooded with passion for my wife and for the close proximity of parenthood, the trust required to take the big step we were about to take together. I knew right then, for the fourth time in my life, I wanted to be a father.

I wanted to raise the child I could have been, to see what I could have achieved had there never been the 5XL shirts and the cruel classmates, like arrogant Wes Simons, who blew elephant noises whenever I walked down the hall.

I wanted something better for something that would be a part of me, and the box at hand was to be the first page of my well-received sequel.

My nine-year-old, size ten feet were locked in exam stirrups, and I was pushing a faux baby out of my faux vagina the first time I knew I wanted to be a father. Mrs. Cole had sent me to the nurse's office for a "bad" cough, a whoop stirred to dramatic effect by purposely constricting the back of my throat until a gravely rattle emerged. What can I say? Third grade was dull, and long division was a rudimentary skill I had taught myself on the front porch three years before. Shivering and scribbling at the old school desk next to my parents' front door, my kindergarten brain deduced the rules of dividing quadruple-digit numbers by double-digit numbers during an early autumn cold spell. A work-fast-or-freeze mentality had taught me in two hours what Mrs. Cole had been scribbling on the chalkboard for over a week, and my phony cough was my last-ditch effort to escape boredom. Angie and April, like any older sisters worth their sinister salt, would lock me outside with their homework and refuse to unlock the door until I had completed my by-proxy assignments, or until Mom and Dad were due home from work. They were only four and five years older than me, but their seemingly innate desire to escape me, to keep their fat brother at arm's length, was advanced passive aggression even for freshly pimpled adolescents.

Mom and Aunt Dee picked me up from school the day of my phony cough and drove me to what had become a monthly appointment at Mercy Medical Clinic in Indianola for both the myriad illnesses I couldn't combat and those I didn't even contract. Construction had finally ceased on the new facility, and the rows of plush chairs and separate television stations, three in all, were far more engaging than repeat lessons on how to dissect simple numbers I already knew how to divvy up. My time was better spent feigning illness and catching up on the latest *All My Children* plot twist.

Every time my name echoed throughout that waiting room, shouted by frumpy Nurse Fat Meanie—an obese Wilma Flintstone look-alike whose girth and oversize trousers were in close competition with my own—my throat constricted. Waves of nausea rushed from my toes, through my stomach, and into the back of my throat. I was burdened with a butter-fly sanctuary that had been in my stomach since birth, and the only way I could keep my recently devoured bag of Doritos from covering Nurse Fat Meanie's sensible shoes was to close my eyes, suck in breath after breath, and hope that the scale measured a smaller number than the last time I had stepped on it. A deep-rooted scale phobia had emerged since a rather demoralizing gym class incident and had only worsened with each notch added to my oversize belt.

Two hundred and sixteen pounds. Up another fourteen pounds since the beginning of third grade when Mr. Osborne, our slightly chubby thirty-something gym teacher, weighed my entire class during gym and the row of stick figures shouted taunts of "Matty Fatty" in a straight, thin line behind me.

"Two hundred and two pounds," he'd whispered, lowering his voice just enough so nobody could hear the number that was three times as large as the weights every other student would hear after stepping down from the scale. "That's what I weigh, big boy." Mr. Osborne's intent could have been an inspirational weight-loss challenge or merely an exasperated commentary in regard to my ill health. But regardless of his intention, the singular outcome was the sick stomach threatening to unload its contents on Nurse Fat Meanie.

"You can have a seat here on the table. Dr. Jasper will be with you shortly," Nurse Fat Meanie said, concealing a smile I knew was her quiet way of celebrating the fact that her personal scale number now was smaller than mine. Come spring weigh-in, Mr. Osborne would do the same.

I hopped up onto the exam table and percussively kicked my legs against the metal frame in a two-step rockabilly beat.

"I swear, that nurse is a real witch with a 'b' every time we come in here," Mom said. "I'm not sure what crawled up her butt and died, but it must have been pretty big."

We all laughed the same voluminous cackle that my mom and her sister had inherited from their father. I had learned to mimic it in order to be one of the gang. I laughed because hearing my mom speak so candidly was like being afforded the freedom to claim a stool at the Corner Tavern and crack open a beer. More important, laughing freed me from feeling like the only one in the barn-style office building who was currently the butt of a fat joke. I needed them to laugh again. I wanted to bury my weight further underground—to keep the good times rolling in order to make the bad ones obsolete.

Between my legs I spotted the black tips of the stirrups jutting out of the table, and in them I discovered my golden ticket to freedom. At first I rubbed my calves with the soft cotton lining of my black jogging pants, a soothing gesture to bide time until the courage arose to pull them out and begin my routine.

Size-ten shoes barely squeezed into the dainty heel slots, but when I was securely fastened, I shoved my legs out to extend the stirrups to a proper distance. My head thrown back, I began to moan.

"Oh, my god, it hurts so bad. Why did you do this to me?" I screamed at the invisible husband at my side, whom I imagined looked like a cross between Harrison Ford and Dave from *Alvin and the Chipmunks*. Soap opera–filled summers provided me ample direction, the dramatic guidance necessary for my first public birthing, and so far my hastily executed plan was succeeding. "I need ice chips! Where are the ice chips? Oh no, another contraction is coming!"

"Matthew, quiet down," Mom laughed, her eyes brimming with tears and her voice quivering with the very distraction I craved. Aunt Dee's laughter was fierce, turning silent at its peak as her bleach blond hair shook like a head-banging lead singer in an eighties metal band. Our fevered, piercing joy was cacophonous and rowdy, an entire studio audience in three bodies, and we never heard the perfunctory knock on the door that announced Dr. Jasper's arrival. Midpush, just as my contractions were at their peak, he walked in the door to find two grown women crying and a ten-year-old boy pretending that the baby inside of him had just crowned.

"Uh, hello again, Matthew," he said. "What seems to be the problem today?"

"I have a cough," I said, frozen in the stirrups, unable to shade the mischief I had created. "I'm not really having a baby."

"Well, that is a relief," he said, placing the earbuds of his stethoscope into his hairy canals. I pushed the stirrups back into the table and sat up straight, ripping the white paper lining on the table as I slid across its surface. "Why don't you lift up your shirt for me so I can listen to your lungs."

Later, on the drive home, Aunt Dee and I both drank orange sodas and sang along to the oldies station while Mom drove the Chevette back to Peru. Nothing blocked my lungs, no strep throat or bronchitis, but I did have another ear infection. My third in as many months.

"You know, you're going to make a great dad someday, Matthew," Mom said. "You're already ready for the birth part of it!"

"Oh, Joy," Aunt Dee said, slapping my mom's arm like girlfriends on TV always did. "You sure are gonna be a great dad, buddy. You are such a good kid. You are going to make someone very, very lucky."

"I can't wait to be a dad," I said. "I love kids."

"Well, please, at least wait until you're eighteen," Mom said, turning up the volume on the stereo, allowing Karen Carpenter's silken voice to change the subject before it veered into reproductive specifics.

⌇⌇⌇

Constance folded the plastic-encased quilt and valance back into the box and tucked the corners, opposite side to opposite side, one under the other, to seal it shut. We hadn't moved from the landing at the top of the stairs since opening the package. Impatience overrode the call for more comfortable amenities once the ogling farmyard animals, flexing their innocent eyes like intimidating biceps, made eye contact with two suckers such as we.

"I love that the animals are raised up," Constance said. "It's even cooler than I thought it would be."

"Me, too. I think the cow is by far the best," I said. "So what do you think we should do with it all now?"

"I guess we'll just put it in the basement until we need it. We don't really have room for it in a closet up here."

"When exactly do you think we'll need it?" I asked. "Sooner rather than later would be pretty cool. I'm excited to decorate the room. To paint and organize the music collection."

One lesser stipulation for pregnancy was to create enough room for baby to exist in what now amounted to a superfluous music room. Three thousand compact discs had to be edited down to a more manageable number—good-bye, Paula Abdul; till next time, Hootie and the Blowfish—and then placed into large, compact carrying cases. With a baby around, there would be no room for the full-size dresser with the sole function of housing my alphabetical glut of CD cases.

"Baby will be soon, Matty, but I do want to finish paying off the debt. We set that as a goal, and I really want to hold to that before we start trying."

"I'm getting so excited, but I also know that's the right thing to do," I said. Lifting the box off the floor, I placed a playful peck on the lid and began walking toward the back door. Out of sight, out of mind.

"Off you go to the basement for now, baby," I said. "See you in four to six months."

Chapter 4

· ·

Pills, Parents, and the Revenge of the Noodle Club

Mom was only nineteen when she gave birth to Angie, and with two months to spare before her twenty-first birthday, she gave birth to her second child, April. By the time I was born—her third and final child conceived by accident and created in the doldrums of a dull Iowa winter—Mom had yet to turn twenty-four. Angie in turn, when she was nineteen, gave birth to Chelsey, and April was twenty-one when she gave birth to Kaela and twenty-four when her second, Ryan, was born.

Constance and I were woefully behind schedule according to the Miller calendar of conception. Married when she was twenty-four and I was twenty-three, we had been bound in matrimony for nearly four years by the time we tossed the plastic birth control wheel into the stainless-steel garbage can.

"Whoa, should we maybe keep that?" I asked. "I mean, I don't think it'll go bad. You'll need it again someday."

"Eh, I'll just get a new one. It's like two bucks with our insurance," Constance said.

Pink tweezers were squeezed between her short fingers, yanking unwanted hairs from above her left eye as she bowed closer and closer toward the mirror until her breath began to fog the glass. "I can't believe I'm not going to be taking that pill. I've taken it every day for over ten years. It blows my mind that we will be having sex without protection."

"Are you nervous?" I asked as I walked over to the trash can and plucked the pink octagon from a bed of discarded tissues and Q-tips. "Just in case. Don't want to accidentally put the kitties on birth control," I lied. Waste annoyed me, even justified waste like stale cookies and leftover pills. I wanted to justify the money we spent on the pills by keeping them tucked inside our green medicine basket just in case Constance changed her mind.

Having babies is no small decision, and I half expected her to jilt our resolution with one decree about the lack of savings in our account, or space in our apartment, or even a suddenly pertinent ten-pound weight-loss goal that would take another month or two to accomplish. Our debt was done, our time off almost banked and secure, and the only thing keeping us from having a baby were the pills I held in my hand.

I dropped the pills back into the garbage can and pushed them underneath the preexisting cotton detritus. No safety blanket, no turning back—the control was now ours.

"No, I'm not nervous," she said. "More scared, I guess. Being pregnant kind of scares me, but I'm ready. And you?"

"I'm not nervous at all," I said. "Actually, I think it's pretty hot."

"You think having unprotected sex is hot?" Constance turned away from the mirror, grabbed the back of my hand, and moved it down over her left breast.

"Yeah, actually, I think it's almost like having sex with a virgin," I said. "Which I never understood what the big deal is about that. I think that's kind of gross with all the blood and pain and whatever. But sex without protection is pretty hot in the same way frat boys think having sex with a virgin is cool. It certainly falls in that category." I gave her breast a playful squeeze and began to slide my hand to the other side of her chest. Before I could make it to the other side, Constance tossed my hand aside, swung around, and dove back into plucking.

"Well, whatever you do, don't tell our kids that," she said. Her eyes greeted mine in the mirror, at first fixed with a serious tone that dissolved into playfulness with a wink. "There's a lot of things we shouldn't tell our kids that we've done."

"Let's go do something right now that we shouldn't tell our kids about," I said, plucking the tweezers from her hand and digging my nose into her neck. I sniffed her clean-scented skin that somehow seemed even paler and more tender than usual. Motherhood already looked good on her, illuminating her with a carefree glow I hadn't seen since we were necking on the dance floor at the Union Bar in Iowa City, grinding our collegiate bodies to overproduced dance music and getting drunk on Jose Cuervo. "You look so beautiful. I love you so much."

Constance turned around and popped up on her tiptoes, elevating herself from an eye-level encounter with my breast-bone to an intimate kiss planted on the side of my neck.

"I love you so much, Matty. I can't wait to have a baby that looks just like you."

"That'll be an awfully big baby," I said, dividing each word into a single statement uttered between kisses that connected the dots of her freckled face. "But it will most likely be bald. I hope it has hair someday, and your blue eyes. You have the most beautiful eyes."

"I hope it has your long legs instead of my short squatty ones."

"I love your short, little legs," I said, tugging the waistband of her fuzzy drawstring pants down past the middle of her limegreen underwear.

"Let's go to the bedroom and get started already," Constance said, putting my index finger against her lips, kissing it, and then placing it in her palm, squeezing me as if looking for relief, pulsing her hand against mine as she dragged me by my digit down the hallway and into the bedroom.

Our decision to start trying was organic and arrived without an excess of words, which was unusual for two nonstop conversationalists such as we. One day the debt was gone: we electronically submitted the final nine-hundred-dollar installment, and we were free. Sushi was our celebration, and as we dipped maki after maki, salmon, scallop, and tuna, we focused on how few people could have razed a five-digit mountain, turning it into ground ready for upward construction in less than two years.

"I guess we should get in touch with Wendy, huh?" Constance asked. "We should start saving money as soon as possible. Start that money market account she was talking about for baby."

"Yeah, I guess so," I said. "It will be nice to start paying ourselves and really nice now that this means we can start trying for a baby soon."

"Well, we can't until June, because that is when I'll finally have enough time to cover all of the leave."

"Oh, yeah, that's right," I said. "For some reason I forgot about that." It was April, and we still had a couple of mistakes to fix on our credit reports, too. Attempting to fix our debt while in Los Angeles, I turned our problems over to a consolidation firm, which then paid three of our credit card bills late and lowered our credit scores.

My eagerness superseded Constance's, but her rationality superseded mine, and June was the compromise we had come up with. I wanted to start sooner, she wanted to start later, and the two markers we set as goals were our best compromise. Constance was still nervous about what a baby would do to her body, to our lives, and to our financial situation, but I didn't care. I was willing to curb cable and trips to Target if it meant we had something that was truly ours, not another immaterial frivolity.

Something in me had snapped when the nursery set arrived. I was an angry suburban wife running over her cheating husband with a Hummer, trapped in a circular zone where the only option that made any sense was to keep driving. I worked as an editor for Content That Works, a newspaper syndicate, and my sudden baby myopia infiltrated every aspect of my job. I assigned health and fitness stories about staying fit during pregnancy and why it is crucial to keep your infant out of eye range and earshot of the television. I assigned home-decorating stories about the hottest trends in nurseries and how Shrek and SpongeBob SquarePants had influenced the current color palette of children's rooms. During lunch with my colleagues Jenn Goebel and Mary Connors, I picked their brains about how altered their lives had become once kids entered the fray.

"It changes everything," Jenn said. "You have no idea how little free time you're going to have or how much patience you're not going to have, but it is all worth it."

"You can't really know until you do it," Mary said. "But

once you do it, it's an overwhelming thing, and you suddenly find yourself thinking, *I can't believe I'm allowed to be a parent. Who am I?* But you do it, and you make it work. It's a remarkably strange thing."

When June finally arrived, and the second pay period of the month officially bestowed Constance with twelve weeks of time off, we sat around the dining-room table with a bottle of pinot noir and a red-pepper frittata coated in goat cheese and caramelized onions—a foodie celebration for what would be a dwindling number of couples-only nights in our future. Mary and Jenn had struck a chord in me, and since our lunch, a melodious ring filled my head that made it seem normal to even want to give up the limitless selfishness of my current state of being so I could be a father. I was eager for the remarkable strangeness of fatherhood.

"I can't believe we're doing this," Constance said, lifting her glass to her lips before we had a chance to toast.

"I can't believe it's finally here," I said, raising my wine glass into the air and holding my arm steady until Constance raised her glass and tapped it against mine. "To what comes next."

"To what comes next."

⤚～⤙

"So, I have some news," I said quietly to my parents into the receiver of our landline phone, which was used primarily to curb the unwanted advances of telemarketers and to order pies we didn't need from the Art of Pizza. Nobody elected to call us at home because we never answered the phone, and I had yet to set up our online voicemail account. Our friends and family gave up trying to reach us on a line that would only ring, leaving them with no other option than to hang up and try again later.

During that particular phone conversation, Mom, Dad, and I had already talked about the weather, my sisters, nieces, nephews, and grandparents. We talked about the torrid pace of new construction, which had forced my dad to work two consecutive weeks of twelve-hour days, stringing ducts along basement ceilings in endless silver trains to drive new furnaces and air conditioners for soon-to-be new homeowners. Mom's work was always fine—never good, never bad, just fine—which often made me wonder if working in insurance was her only way to ascertain insurance coverage and stock her savings for a thirteen-gift-per-person-minimum Christmas celebrations.

Erring on the side of timidity, I had held off telling my parents about our decision for two weeks. Procreation was nothing to joke about in my family whose children are fireworks on the Fourth of July, and every explosion elicits cheers, tears, and congratulations and, soon thereafter, calls for the next one to ignite. Sex wasn't something I talked about with my parents, either. Dad never told me two words about my penis. Mom never gave me guidance about the ins and outs of the vagina.

Had it not been for life in a small town, which drove my neighbor Rachel and me to early exploration, I very easily could have made it to high-school health class before I learned that my penis did more than pee.

Sex was not an open topic in our house unless it was part of a joke. The one exception was the time Dad found a pornographic video in my VCR during my senior year of high school. He went in to watch a taped performance of his band's latest performance in my bedroom while Mom watched a romantic comedy on the big screen. When I came home from the movies with my buddy, Orion, Dad told me nothing like that was allowed in the house again, then made me take it out to my Mustang right then and there. *Guns and Hoses* was never to be spoken of again.

And even though this time would be different because the sex I was alluding to would lead to a baby, my reticence was a Pavlovian reflex.

"Tell them," Constance whispered, pacing around the kitchen while I sat on the counter stabbing a serrated knife into an apple that I planned to eat as soon as I broke the news and ended the conversation.

"That's really great, Dad," I said. He had installed two geo-furnaces in two and a half days, which had bought him enough time to finish hooking up eight air conditioners by the end of the day. "So, uh, I have some news."

"What's that, Matthew?" Mom asked.

"Well, it's nothing yet, but Constance and I have decided to start trying for a baby," I said, poking the knife all the way through the apple and into the wooden countertop beneath.

"Oh, Matthew, that's so great!" Mom said.

"Congratulations, buddy," Dad said. "We wondered when you guys were going to have one. I told your mom it would be soon. Looks like you made your mom cry. You know how sensitive she is."

I explained to them the situation without outlining more than a line-item litany of our reasons. Debt details would have depressed my parents, who never had a credit card of their own, save for Mom's JC Penney account. Angie's ex-husband had single-handedly tanked their credit and racked up thousands in debt, and I had been within earshot to hear Dad wax on about the "moron" it takes to buy into credit-card schemes. So I focused on the positives, about how I wanted to finish my master's thesis, how we wanted to "get our finances in order," how we wanted to have ample time together as a married couple, and how Constance wanted to save up enough leave to take three full months off after the baby was born.

"You guys are very responsible," Dad said. "There's no rush to these sorts of things. You gotta do what you gotta do."

"So, yeah, I'm very excited," I said, removing the knife from the apple and taking a taste in midsentence. My first bite was sweet, and the flesh of the apple was crisper than I'd expected. "Excuse my apple, I'm just so stoked about this I've gotta eat something."

"I can't wait to tell everybody," Mom said. "Is it okay if I tell everybody?"

"Absolutely," I said. "Are you excited to be a grandma again?"

~~~

"Why are you telling me this?" Susan asked. "I mean I'm happy for you, but it sems like this is something you don't need to tell me. Don't people just do it?"

"I don't know, I guess because it was a huge decision for us, and I thought you'd be excited that your only daughter was ready to have a baby," Constance said, pounding her free hand against an invisible wall, driving a nail through her mother's thick-walled response. Constance pulled her cell phone away from her ear and covered the mouthpiece. "Can you believe this?" she mouthed to me, rolling her eyes in never-ending circles and forcing the deflation of her expectations with a succession of elongated breaths.

"Well, I'm sorry to have bothered you while you were out with your friends, Mom. I guess I'll just let you go."

Susan was out shopping with the women from her noodle club in Pinehurst, North Carolina. Once a week the women of the noodle club would drive an SUV to the lakefront, dive into the human-made body of water surrounded by curving lines of unconscionably large homes, and float for two hours with the aid of Styrofoam noodles. Exercise was the goal, but conversation was the only outcome. Constance was anxious to share a genuine mother-daughter moment, a rare gender-specific bond between a feminist and an upper-crust etiquette maven living half a country away. Following a trip to her gynecologist, Constance officially had been flashed a baby-making green light and our car was not only in gear, but barreling down the freeway at dangerously high velocities. Catching her parents up-to-speed felt as natural of a next step as painting the walls a neutral sage green in the third bedroom earmarked for baby.

Susan believed our casual confession was a bit gauche and confusing. A woman didn't need to call her mother to relay such a personal topic, especially since there was no news to report. Emily Post would find it in poor taste to e-mail a thank-you card, and she certainly wouldn't approve of a carefree, preconception dialogue between mother and child in the middle of the afternoon—or so it seemed to Constance.

"She was laughing at me," Constance said. "She was with her friends and started making such a condescending fuss about how silly my call was. It was really insulting."

"That's crap," I said, grabbing her by the upper arms and spinning her around, placing her shoulders into the nook between my pecs for an impromptu massage. Sunlight was spiraling through the Coke-glass window behind the fridge, filling the room with a rainstorm of dust particles. I closed my eyes to keep out both the light and the dust, and blindly kneaded Constance's shoulders. "Your mom is so unpredictable. I would have thought she'd be sky high right now at the prospect of her only child having a baby."

"Me, too," she quivered, her words shaped into a lonely aria by a vibrato of swallowed embarrassment. News of our decision was personal, and we had refrained from telling anyone but our parents. I got to have my moment, the initial celebration of generational expansion between parents and a child, but Constance felt slighted on her first chance to share the joy.

Forty-five minutes later, after we'd made love in the absence of affirmation to reclaim the tenderness of our decision, the phone vibrated across the bedside table and clinked against the glass water carafe like the prongs of a fork colliding with teeth.

"It's my mom," Constance said.

"Don't answer it," I said, moving my hand to her forehead to sweep misdirected curls out of her eyes. "Just let it go to voicemail and let her stew for a little bit. She's earned herself some time in the noose."

"No, I should answer it." Constance flipped open the phone and wiggled her body back and forth until she was seated upright, still tucked between the purple flower-print Calvin Klein sheets. "Hi, Mom. What's up?" she asked, propping three pillows behind her back to soften her stance against the sturdy wood headboard. "That's okay. I was just surprised you acted that way. We thought you'd be happy and not mean."

Susan polled her noodle-club buddies, and when the other women confessed that their daughters had done or would make the identical phone call, that any mother would be thrilled to receive word that her daughter was ready to continue the cycle they started, it dawned on her that the only action worthy of being deemed inappropriate was her reaction.

"It's okay. It was a mistake. We're just really excited about having a baby and wanted to share the news."

Constance told her mom about the nursery set boxed in the basement, her clean bill of health, and the dead debt we buried less than a month ago.

"Thanks, Mom. I'm pretty proud of us, too," Constance said, leaning her head against my chest and writhing her fingers through the dense hair. She began to stroke the air above my shoulder, patting an imaginary head and rubbing an imaginary backside that would have extended down to my ribs. Lying in bed, we had begun to practice what it would be like to have a child between our bodies, on our stomachs, or wrapped in our arms. Now that our parents knew our intentions, the imaginary baby we conjured in our bed felt a little more real and a little less like a psychotic playtime shared by two. Our baby was closer now than ever before. Telling her parents had constructed a roadblock that, to turn back now, would allow their guilt to guilt us into staying the course or at least put us to bed without dinner for being so irresponsible.

I was no longer the kid who called for a ride home on the second day of camp because I smelled like death and the public showers were too humiliating for a fat boy to face. I finally had become a father, and to be afraid of the public nudity, my scarred body, or a baby now felt unnecessary. I finally had a reason to be me with no apologies and no regrets.

Chapter 5

· ·

Baby, Baby, and
Two More Babies

"I'm pregnant," she said, her voice quivering with a disbelief I'd heard only in the voices of grateful hurricane survivors and camera-shy lotto winners on CNN. "I can't believe it finally happened. I was so shocked that I took three pregnancy tests and all of them were positive."

Rocks cluttered the sidewalk along Montrose Avenue as late-summer construction workers tore up every street corner for miles, leaving piles of jagged concrete stacked like abandoned games of prehistoric Tetris. My manicured beard scratched against the receiver of my cell phone and each step along the rocky terrain muffled my excitement.

"I'm stunned into silence," I said. "Honestly, I never ever thought that would happen. I never thought we'd get to have this conversation today or any other day. It's been so long in coming." Eyes burning from a mix of pollen and jealousy, I paused to take a deep breath, deep enough to push the emotions far enough away to muster a "I'm so excited, Angie. I'm so happy for you."

Walking was initiated by an email that popped up in my inbox around eight forty-five AM, before I'd had a chance to finish making the rounds to my favorite music websites (which always preceded diving into a wreckage of edits, photos, and writing assignments that dripped onto my schedule from the previous day's to-do list). ARE YOU READY TO BE AN UNCLE AGAIN? was the subject line, and to my amazement, the sender was not my sister who still had a complete cervix.

Angie had given birth to Chelsey fourteen years ago, three days before my last day of junior high school. A couple of years later, some precancerous polyps were discovered during a routine exam, and over half of her cervix had to be removed to ensure cancer would not advance. After Angie remarried a much nicer man with a son of his own, the newlyweds tried and tried to conceive, to create a shared life, but her doctors said the chances of conception, or at least a pregnancy that could endure without much of a cervix, would almost be impossible.

Ten years of trying, and it finally happened for her, and as I increased the pace at which I walked down the street in an effort to break a sweat and break down my jealousy, I allowed her disbelief to fuel my support.

"I made Junior run out for a second package of tests because it couldn't be real. The medicine I'm on to regulate my periods makes it so I have to take a pregnancy test every month to make sure I'm not pregnant, and for ten years it has been negative. Matty, I never thought this would happen."

Angie and Junior even had considered adopting a Chinese girl, an idea to which my dad was less than amenable. Even more than his parental discontent—my father's disbelief that Angie could love an adopted child with a ferocity equal to her love for true lineage—it was the crashing waves of irrepressible loss that drowned my sister. To give up hope that one day she could have a child with the man she truly loved would be an "end" where a "start" should have existed.

"Will there be complications?" I asked, plugging my left ear as jackhammers pounded a tribal beat in cadence with my pace, which had quickened in coordination with my escalating excitement. Welles Park was straight ahead, and I knew that at this time on a summer day children and parents would be on blankets, filling the baseball outfield adjacent to Sulzer Library. It seemed like a proper setting to revel in her news.

"I have to go in for a lot of checkups, but my doctor is hopeful. They just have to monitor me very closely."

A free bench at the south end of the park was cluttered with single pages of the *Chicago Tribune* waving in the scream-filled breeze as countless children ran circles in the grass. Parents on cell phones, noses in books, babies on blankets, toddlers running parallel to traffic barricaded by a black steel fence, and my sister finally pregnant again. All was as it should have been.

"It'll be so nice for our kid to have a cousin its own age," I said, pushing aside news of the latest Cubs loss to make room to sit. "Constance and I were talking about that just the other day, about how old all the other kids in our family will be compared to ours. It's so cool he or she will have a playmate."

"It'll happen for you soon, Matty. Sometimes it just takes time. It's only been two months."

After hanging up with my sister, her voice a thin, uncertain breath, I dialed Constance to break the news. Before I could say a word, though, she began to speak.

"Matty, guess who's pregnant?"

"That's weird," I said, "I was going to ask you the exact same thing."

"Me first," she said. "It's somebody we met in Chicago."

"Krista?"

"Matty, be serious."

"What? Lesbians can have babies." Two women speed-walking strollers shot lasers of disapproval toward me, either afraid that due to my influences their infants would soon begin questioning the origins of the word *lesbian* or themselves lesbians assuming my words were derogatory.

"But Krista obviously didn't just happen to get pregnant. We would have known that ahead of time."

"Then I have no idea."

"Come on, just guess."

"Okay . . . is it Cathy?"

"How did you know?"

"Well, I knew by your tone it had to be shocking, and she's the dumbest person I've ever met. Seemed like a logical leap. I mean she is a dumb, dumb woman." Another mother pushing a stroller, a pink headband pushing a lick of red curls into a poof on top of her head, had stopped next to my bench to tie her shoe. She shot me a second fierce look as I admonished a woman she didn't even know. Sensitive ears abounded in a park that was not a safe place for my racy candor, so I vacated my bench and began the six-block walk back to my office.

"On a separate note, somebody told me at work that I was the next one in line to have a baby. Can you believe that? That kind of shit makes me so angry. For all they know I can't have kids. Or don't want kids."

"Yeah, the assumptions are rotten. For all they know I'm really a barren woman and you're my disgruntled cross-dressing husband." This time it was a jogger slowing up as he passed me, cranking his head over his right shoulder and scrunching his face like a troll. I turned my head to deflect his disapproving gaze with a shrug and an inappropriately wide grin. "You just never know, and when you don't know, you should just shut up."

"But at the same time I wanted that to be me," Constance said, skipping stones over my third attempt to lighten the moment. "I wanted to be the one announcing that. Where's our baby?"

"I don't know, baby. We haven't been trying for that long. But speaking of trying for a long time, I actually do have some funny news. We aren't even going to be the next people to announce a pregnancy in my family."

"April's pregnant?"

"Nope. April has her tubes tied. It's Angie."

"What? I don't understand. I thought she couldn't have any more kids with the cervix thing."

"It's a medical miracle, I guess. She sounds shell-shocked. I just can't stop smiling. That's going to be one lucky kid, though. She and Junior are going to make wonderful parents. They are such calm people, and they have their lives and finances together. It's going to be such a different experience than her first time around."

Silence pulsed on the line, and without a word, without an explanation for the space in between my words and this moment, I knew Constance couldn't say the word *jealousy* despite being buried beneath an avalanche of green.

"I'm so happy for her," Constance said thirty seconds later, her voice a half octave lower and four notches softer than at the beginning of our chat. "I mean, she's wanted that forever, but it's so hard to hear about everybody else getting pregnant and not feel this way."

This way she was feeling never attached itself to a word,

but as I climbed the dark, industrial staircase back into my office and closed my cell phone to end the conversation, the elation I felt on behalf of my sister was tempered with a bit of the same, unspoken emotion.

Chapter 6

· ·

Periods, Parties,
and Something That Was Nothing

Blood arrived on cue twenty-eight days after the previous month's menstruation had faded into skyline pink and disappeared completely. Standing over Constance's shoulder to monitor her maxi pad while she sat on the toilet was a new addition to our accepted coupling activities, but one I knew would be only momentary.

No amount of premarital brainstorming about the first moment the possibility of pregnancy entered our relationship would have placed me in my current situation, locked in the cockpit, helicoptering over my wife's feminine hygiene routine, hoping her preemptively applied maxi pad would remain as white as it had been while encapsulated in the translucent blue plastic. But the prospect that she would pull down her pants and reveal only a blank canvas, an untainted cotton butterfly that would speak volumes of my virility, was too irresistible for me to avoid. Merv Griffin couldn't have created a more compelling game show than *Pregnant/Not Pregnant?*—a game of chance where every trip to the bathroom brings you closer to pregnancy or closer to devastation.

"Well, so much for that," Constance said, standing up from the toilet and washing her hands. "Maybe in October."

"Eh, it's only been three months," I said, walking out of the bathroom and into the kitchen. "Mom says it can take time for all of those years of birth control to get out of your system."

"Three to six months is what I read," Constance said. "It's so funny though, 'cuz I always thought the first time I had sex without using the pill I would get pregnant. As irrational as I know that is, it was engrained in me that unprotected sex equals pregnancy."

"Yeah, I know it's pretty unlikely, but I thought we had a good chance of getting pregnant the first month. My whole life I've just felt so fertile."

"Me, too!" she shrieked, pulling open the refrigerator door and removing a carton of orange juice from between two rows of diet soda. "I was terrified all of the way through college that I would get pregnant before I had my life together. I had such a clear plan to get my undergraduate degree, my master's, and then get a kick-ass job. After that I would wait until I was thirty-two and either have a baby or adopt, depending on if I was married or not."

"Every person in my family gets pregnant at the drop of a hat," I said, grabbing a protein bar from the pantry shelf in an effort to boost my postrun energy and, subconsciously, to complete a masculine task in light of our failure. "I mean, seriously, the men and women on both sides of my family were born to breed and eat ice cream. We're not just your run-of-the-mill fertile people; we're exceptionally skilled at fertility. We are to fertility what Tiger Woods is to upscale product endorsements."

"Well, I'm sure it will happen soon enough," Constance said, swirling the dregs of the juice that clung to the sides and bottom of her glass, sucking the last bits from the rim as if she were nursing an empty bottle, with her pouty, plump lips—lips I hope would be passed on to our daughter in lieu of my unassuming, unspectacular pair.

Those were the lips that would negotiate later curfews, higher allowances, and forgiveness in the face of dented fenders and exorbitant text-message overages. Those were the lips I loved to kiss, and I was immediately reminded that there remained a magnitude of good things about childlessness.

"Well, that's just one more month I get you all to myself," I said, wrapping my arms around her, the glass still clutched in her hand. Waddling side to side, she was the pendulum of a clock and I moved with her in time.

"Ah, I don't know what to do with my glass," Constance said, wriggling free from my embrace and laughing with me at her own expense. "But honestly, Matty, that is a great thing. More time with you is all I ever want. That's the greatest gift I could get."

~⸲~

Month four swept by with nothing more than waiting to mark the time. In an effort to demarcate the first trimester of trying from the unforeseeable future, to lock our unborn failures in the trunk and drive our broken-down car into Lake Michigan, we decided what we most needed was to get unruly drunk. More specifically, I needed to drink copious amounts of red wine and dance until I passed out, or at least until I whetted my prebaby drought with the irresponsibility of a late night and the overindulgence of off-limits food and drink.

E-vites were distributed for Matt & Constance's 1st Ever Annual Wine, Chocolate, and Cheese party, urging our guests to get their Starbucks on and their J-Crew out of the closet for a night of unadulterated frivolity. October 7, 2006, was chosen because it was one day after Constance's period was due, which allowed us to know going into the evening of debauchery whether or not we could debauch with our guests. We had yet to tell anyone except our parents about our decision to have a baby, and nowhere on the invitations did it hint at a deeper need than upscale escapism.

"Peeing on the stick is best in the morning," Constance said. "I'll do it first thing when I wake up."

"What do you mean it's best in the morning?" I asked.

"Apparently your pee has the largest concentration of baby hormones in the morning."

"Not my pee."

"No, Matty. Not your pee," Constance said, patting my back as if I were a toddler who had just proven my ability to pee in the toilet for the first time. Before bed we walked to CVS to buy a two-pack of tests and a pint of vanilla ice cream.

Constance and I recently had discovered our inner craftiness was capable of greatness, and that greatness had ascended to the creation of homemade marshmallows and graham crackers, which would serve as the s'mores-making centerpiece of the chocolate table. We spent the entire day of the party whipping gelatin and water into fluff before placing it in foil-lined pans until time had turned the concoction into marshmallows. It was a squishy, pure sugar antidote to remove our minds from the single line. A single line so distinct and lonely no amount of time spent staring at its singularity could coax a second line to appear.

Our guests arrived, dressed to the yuppie nines, each bearing a bottle of their favorite wine, a bar of chocolate, and a block of cheese. The table was lined with fresh baguettes and signs to label each food with a literary moniker. Graham Greene Crackers and Somerset Maughamallows mingled with Catcher in the Rye Bread, For Whom the Brie Tolls, and Like Water for 88% Dark Chocolate. Mary Fons, one of my childhood best friends who also found her second life in Chicago, arrived fashionably late dressed in black-and-white business attire, an attaché case in one hand and a Venti Latte in the other.

"I just flew in from New York this morning after a meeting with Marty and simply had to grab a nonfat sugar-free vanilla caramel latte, hold the cream, before I could do one more thing," she joked, hugging me only with her torso, pressing her props into my back.

Twelve wine bottles later, the crowd gathered in the living room. Mary performed selections from her slam poetry oeuvre with the partygoers gathered around her feet as if she were the leader of our nonrhyming resistance. Constance and I sat on the sofa, sipping pinot noir and holding hands, and I couldn't stop my mind from dancing right into the arms of guilt that had squeezed me daily since we began trying.

What if this was the month? What if we finally managed to get sperm to the egg and our firstborn child was conceived via two systems raging with tannins and alcohol? What if the pregnancy test was wrong? What if our only child was born with two eyes sprouting out of the center of his or her face because mommy and daddy needed a juvenile drunken break from the pressures of fruitless sex? As the crowd erupted into applause, with Mary graciously bowing, hands pressed together in grateful praise, I looked over at Constance and forced a cautious smile despite the disfigured babies dancing in my head to the cadence of my guests' colliding hands. Her blue eyes rolled lazily in her head, and her cheeks were flushed pink.

"She's so good," Constance said, squeezing my hand. "I really needed that. And this."

"Yeah," I said, "she's a really talented girl and this is a really great party." Mary was a searchlight and her gift for illuminating the obvious cast a glow on Constance's needy face. She needed one night without the caffeine restrictions and vitamins, the regimen recommended for optimum preconception health, and I knew it was what I needed, too. One night would not endow fetal alcohol syndrome upon our child unless the party devolved into raucous rounds of wine bongs, and even then it would likely be a subtle affectation. Fifteen minutes later, Kamila Brodowinska, Jenni Hansen, and I took the stage to perform for the second time as Urgency, my rock band that was destined for greatness. By the time we completed our seven-song set, I was too drunk to comprehend that my guitar stand was about one foot to the left of where I dropped my acoustic electric Dean onto the hardwood floor. I was a nobody version of Keith Richards who had yet to rock hard enough in his life to properly handle his chemical and his axe.

"Let's dance," I yelled, leaving the guitar where it landed until the feedback from the amp worked itself into high-pitched swirls that matched the movement of my head. Jenni picked up my acoustic and placed it into the stand, where I had intended to place it from the outset. "The band that dances together stays together."

Outside on the porch, the smokers had gathered to talk about things only the nicotine dependent and their loved ones who put up with the cold and secondhand toxins ever get to hear. A bond is formed between puffs. In the sharing of lighters, an aura of eventual death and future oxygen-tank dependencies and the formal conventions of pleasantry-filled conversations are eschewed for immediate grit. When Constance disappeared I knew her former smoking habit had lured her to take up residence with Jenni, Kamila, and Mary outdoors.

When I walked out onto the porch, all four women gave me a cockeyed glance replete with half-mouth smiles—looks that come only when you enter a space in which either your sexual prowess or financial status is being discussed without your prior consent.

"Hey, buddy!" Kamila shouted. "You've been going at it pretty hard I hear."

"I told them," Constance said. "I told them about how you have to have sex every day or you get cranky."

"Wow," I said, my face melting into gaunt blankness.

"Well, it's true," she said. "It really is, he's insatiable." Constance directed her comments at the women around her, talking about my bedroom needs as if she were in the throes of the ubiquitous café girl-talk scene in an estrogen-filled Kate Hudson movie.

"All right, buddy," Kamila said.

"We've been trying to get pregnant, but we haven't done it yet," Constance said. "We have sex all the time, and I thought I'd get pregnant the very first time I had unprotected sex, but we're entering the fourth month of trying and nothing yet. Hell, maybe I'm pregnant right now. I should have gotten my period today, but I didn't. We did a test, but it was negative, but it could have just been too soon to test. Wouldn't that be just so like us, Matty? For us to finally be pregnant the one night I'm drinking and smoking?"

"Matty, you never told us you guys were trying to get pregnant," Jenni said, slapping me on the arm just like Constance does when exasperated by my refusal to communicate.

"I, uh, well, we never really told anybody except our parents," I said. "We just kinda thought we'd tell people once we got pregnant, since you never know how long it can take."

"You guys are going to be great parents," Mary said. "And, girl, you just be glad you got a man that can keep up. You go, Matty. Get 'er done."

"Oh, he can keep it up all the time," Constance said. "I swear sometimes that's all he would do if it were up to him."

"I always figured you were one of those guys," Jenni said. "Don't worry, I'm like that, too. Lissette and I could do it every night if it was up to me."

"Okay, I'm going back inside," I said, furrowing my brow and squinting my eyes in an attempt to properly convey both my confusion and discomfort. "I, uh, okay. You guys have fun out here."

The annual Covered Bridge Festival held in Winterset, Iowa, home of my high school and also John Wayne's birthplace, was feted the week following our party a mere three hundred and fifty miles away from Chicago. The coronation of the Winterset Town Square as the go-to spot for fried-pork sandwiches, church pies, jams, honey, and spelling bees was a tired concoction of fat and kitsch, and something the Miller family would miss only under extreme duress. Since leaving home, it had become an impromptu reunion for all of us, minus Dad, who believed the whole event was a thinly veiled attempt to extort money from the good people trying to access the town square's myriad businesses. Upon completion of another dull Friday, our friend Krista and her partner, Cheryl, made the six-hour drive to Iowa with us under the guise of devouring pork tenderloin sandwiches bigger than a human face. We spent the entire journey listening to gimmicky country music about girls in T-shirts downing tequila shots with cowboys, and one-night stands that culminate with the empowered cowgirl riding off in her pickup truck the following morning without so much as a tip of the hat.

"I once sang this song at our eighth-grade talent show," I said as a treble-heavy version of Garth Brooks's "That Summer" crackled through our factory stereo.

"You sang what?" Krista shrieked.

"Yeah, I know, right?"

"You do realize this song is about a teenager and an old farm hag shacking up together," Krista said.

"Oh, yeah," I said. "I wore my black cardigan and navy blue Dockers and belted it out while Mrs. Bechtol rocked the piano. It was a real coming-of-age moment for me."

"Oh, my god, that's the funniest thing I've ever heard," Krista said, forcing words through cracks in her wall of laughter. "I can just see you singing that song and the whole crowd looking so confused."

"I was a soulful boy," I said. "I really sold it."

Tears poured out of Constance's eyes as she sliced the darkness along I-80 with our silver PT Cruiser, wiping her eyes with the sleeve of her brown sweater to keep her vision clear enough to steer.

"You know you're going to have a little Matt that's just like you someday," Cheryl said. "Standing up in front of the entire school to sing a song about bagging some old chick."

"Yeah, your little Garth might be coming very soon," Krista said.

After our party—after a negative pregnancy test and a night of drunkenness—Constance's period never arrived. Sunday came and went, mainly in swirling and pounding strokes with our heads buried beneath pillows and blankets, but the missing period entered its second day of absence.

"If it doesn't come by Wednesday, we'll test again," Constance said on the Monday morning following our party. She applied her professional face—mascara, eyeliner, and eye shadow—while I sat on the floor reading Sunday's *Chicago Tribune* that had gone untouched due to our hangovers. "God, can you even believe that the one time I'm finally late is the one time I drank and smoked in the last six months? Seriously, our baby is going to be deformed, and we will have no one to blame but ourselves."

"Our baby will not be deformed," I said, lowering the local news page to find her eyes in the mirror. "Plenty of people drink one time and have perfectly normal babies. Hell, some people drink frequently and have a perfectly normal baby. Just don't beat yourself up over it."

"But I will beat myself up," Constance said. "I deserve to be beaten up a bit because it was stupid to let my guard down for the night. I just thought for sure that the negative test meant I wasn't pregnant."

Agreeing verbally or mentally wouldn't make the guilt of our alcohol-fueled fun regress, so I grabbed Constance by the shoulders and dug my fingers into her tight shoulders.

Two days later, five days post party, the test once again produced a solitary line, even though the elusive period remained in the shadows. Arrogance blossomed inside of me; I knew our baby was in the midst of cellular division whether or not the test agreed with me. Before leaving work on Friday to begin our road trip, I researched instances when pregnant women didn't test positive on at-home tests.

During our drive to Iowa with Krista and Cheryl, we stood

a full week late, and both of us were reasonably confident that our baby was alive and growing. Placing my hand on Constance's stomach, I rubbed clockwise circles against her flesh and sang a verse of "Losing My Religion" into her gut. My innate music snobbery had overshadowed the wants of the car's other inhabitants, and it was the first song all night that I felt comfortable singing to my future baby.

"We decided if the period doesn't come by the time we get back from Covered Bridge Festival on Monday," Constance said, peeking into the rearview mirror to make eye contact with our passengers, "we'll take one more test and then go to the doctor. Obviously, something is going on." The next morning we woke at dawn and drove our empty stomachs to the festival. Pregnancy was going on; I was sure of it, and as we walked around the town square with steaming apple ciders and baskets of fried brown foods, onion rings indistinguishable from funnel cake, I walked ahead of the pack with my sister Angie and told her the news.

"You know, Cody's wife, Sandy, is pregnant, too," Angie said, pushing through the packs of flannel-outfitted patrons shoving foods on sticks into their mouths as they walked down the middle of the road.

"No, nobody told me that," I said. "Good for them. It would be so cool to have three new babies in the family. It's been such a long time since we've had any new additions." Kids were fixtures on the town square that day, weaving between and around the wooden shacks, pounding on the walls of the miniature likenesses of the famous *Bridges of Madison County* used to sell cheap goods to tourists. Boys twirled plastic guns around their index fingers outside the John Wayne memorabilia booth, standing next to an oversize cardboard blowup of our town's most famous son.

"Mom is gonna go crazy," Angie said. "Her favorite little boy finally giving her another baby to love."

Giving my mom the gift of another grandchild: Angie's suggestion ignited my deep-set eyes with the soft burn of tears, and my usually virile mind, a dictionary of uncomplicated words, forfeited its penchant for never shutting up. Spelling-bee contestants were announcing letters over the loudspeaker in the background, the same spelling bee I won in the fourth grade after throwing up in the port-a-potty because of a nervous stomach. Walking up the steps of the courthouse to exhibit my phonetic dexterity in front of my mom made me too nervous to keep the caramel apple in my stomach. I had always wanted to impress my mom, to give her something for which to be proud of me, and even though I had graduated college and had recently attained my master's degree, I knew that my having a baby was something she wanted for me above all else.

"I don't know if I'm going to tell her until I know for sure," I said. "I don't want to get her hopes up if the tests are right and we're wrong."

"You should tell her something," Angie said, walking out of the John Wayne booth and into a hut filled with stuffed dolls with braids of colored yarn and prairie-style two-pocket dresses. "You know Mom. She probably suspects something is up anyway."

Later that night we went to the old Circle B Cashway lumberyard that had been converted by my cousin's cousin into a country-and-western bar. Dad's cover band, The Drifters, had been entertaining southern Iowa's two-step crowd since 1985, and the annual Covered Bridge Festival dance was a hit-or-miss affair depending on the weather and the number of tourists and locals able to dance with bellies full of batter.

Mom sat next to the soundboard, tweaking knobs, balancing the level, and minimizing the electric guitar, which she usually did to keep herself occupied in bars and dancehalls where nearly everyone was a stranger or a drunk. Krista and I engaged in a spirited waltz around the dance floor, two Amazonian giants circling in an out-of-the-box unison, and when the song stopped, I walked over to my mom and pulled up a second metal folding chair.

"How's it going?" I asked.

"It's good, Matthew," she said. "You looked awfully good out there dancing. Do you remember when we used to dance all the time? You were always such a good little two-stepper."

"You weren't so bad yourself," I said. "And I was so big, people probably thought I was your husband, not your son."

"Oh, Matthew!" Ounces of truth about my excessive weight were always greeted with that exact exasperated emission, even now that I had grown lanky. Since the last time we visited, Mom's thin lips had gathered a new set of wrinkles as a result of losing half of herself on Jenny Craig. Her partially annoyed, partially doting expression now matched the bunched folds of the too-large tan sweater gathered around her waist.

"So, I have some interesting news," I said, sucking the Miller Lite bottle between my lips to buy precious seconds before I dropped the baby bomb and her emotional shrapnel was sent flying into the eyes and ears of every bedazzled cowgirl within earshot.

"What's that?" she asked, placing her hand on my back and scratching an unknown itch that only her parental instincts could have sensed was in need of sharp attention.

"Constance's period is eight days late," I said. "We took two pregnancy tests and both were negative, but she's really late. I've read a lot online about women who don't test positive until their second or third month of pregnancy, so I'm guessing it's just a mistake. We're going to test again Wednesday and then go to the doctor."

No tinny shrieks and no alarming yelps escaped Mom's lips, no deafening adulation or drop-everything embraces, which were the benchmark expectations I had set for the announcement. Instead, puddles of water pooled inside her glassy hazel eyes, which began to stream, single file, down her reddening cheeks as the band began a lyrically inaccurate rendition of "La Bamba."

"Matthew, that is so wonderful," she said, dropping her scratching hand down into mine and squeezing with no regard for the amount of pressure she was placing on the thin, prominent bones of my ten-inch hands. "You guys are going to make such great parents."

"Would you like to two step, for old-time's sake?" I asked, extending my hand in princely fashion to whisk my mom onto the dance floor, the aggressive beat too infectious to ignore despite the guitar player's mangled, offensive attempts to sing in Spanglish. Dad didn't dance and Mom still had the feet and soul of a young woman walking into the gymnasium on prom night.

"I would love to, Matthew," she said, grabbing my hand with a delicate touch, stiffening in expectation that I would lean backward and pull her to her feet. After the song finished, we seamlessly danced into the next four-minute composition before Mom felt obligated to return to the soundboard.

"Thanks," she said, "and I can't wait to hear on Wednesday what you guys find out."

Wednesday morning's first pee hit the stick and, in accordance with the previous two tests, yielded only one pink line. Wednesday's second pee, arriving courtesy of a twenty-four ounce strawberry smoothie only thirty minutes after the first, yielded the first spots of blood from the ten-days-late period.

"I'm not pregnant," Constance said. She sat on the toilet crying into my shoulder for five minutes before starting to rub lotion on her legs, white streaks stroked across her calves waiting to moisturize while we coped with losing something that could have been nothing, but something that had become something over the course of the last two hundred and forty misleading hours. "Will you call your mom and Angie and tell them? I don't want anybody spreading the gossip that we're pregnant. I feel so stupid."

"Me, too," I said, closing my eyes, feeling the ghost of Mom's arm around my waist as we shuffled in honor of nothing. She was so happy, and I was so happy to finally make her so happy. "I'll call them right now."

Chapter 7

· ·

The Second Time I Knew
I Wanted to Be a Father

A rainbow of scattered plastic eggs arced across
the front lawn, which had recently become overgrown with
dandelions and BMX bicycles. My family never celebrated the
resurrection of Jesus by taking to the stiff, oily pews of the Peru
United Methodist Church, nor did we commemorate the
occasion by putting ash on our foreheads and giving up soda
for a month so we would be assured our room in heaven. We
chose to honor a sugar-induced belief that Easter was a celebration of rabbits. More specifically, rabbits who delivered
Hawaiian-print shorts, tennis rackets, and chocolate self-
replicas in pink wicker baskets because no one had burned
down the house or caused bodily harm to another family
member since Santa skipped town in December.

Outside the window, our candy plantation stirred my antic-
ipatory stomach, with hundreds of pastel ovals waiting to be
plucked like ripe pecans aching to find their way into a pie.

Mom was still dressed in her blue cotton nightgown in the kitchen frying sausages, whipping pancake batter, and whistling selections from the Patsy Cline catalog. Angie and her daughter, Chelsey, were still sleeping. Angie never liked to depart bed before the sun hit its peak, and her daughter had followed suit. April wasn't going to leave her dilapidated apartment or her boyfriend to drive forty-five miles for candy she could buy through the bullet-proof walk-up window at the 7-11 two blocks away from her home.

My knees ached as I stood by the window and wondered which of the baskets held my candy. Picking up my roll of stomach fat, I laid it on the wooden windowsill to remove excess pressure from my spine, the extremes of my stomach pulling my shoulders down into a slouch.

"Good morning, buddy," Dad said as he opened the bedroom door. His massive brown-rimmed glasses covered the upper third of his face and sat like an imbalanced teeter-totter across the bridge of his nose. Dad's inevitable cowlick jutted out the back of his head like an oversize price tag. Every morning, he emerged from the bedroom crusty eyed and stumbling, his white hairless belly sagging over his equally white briefs. He walked into the bathroom, uttering a couple of nonsensical words before slamming shut the bathroom door and disappearing for twenty minutes.

I picked up my stomach fat from the windowsill and walked to the sofa to watch television while I waited. At sixteen, I was too old to want this so badly, but I wanted my candy in spite of my age and body aches. My legs throbbed from holding up my weight in one place for ten minutes. I massaged my puffy knees and admired Brad Pitt as he hopped into the back of Thelma and Louise's convertible.

I wish my ass got people's attention like that, I thought, prodding the chub pushing out from the sides of my bones, kneading my fat like wounded dough.

Once the familiar on-cue muskiness of Brut cologne began to waft under the bathroom door, I knew Dad soon would emerge a put-together man. Tugging on the bottom of his Chicago Bears sweatshirt, stretching the fabric to cover his belly, he walked over to my seat on the sofa and extended a hand.

"Come on, buddy, we need to go out and cover the sewer."

"Dad, I want to watch TV. I don't feel like working on the sewer."

"Nope, it's good for you to turn off the television and get outside to do something once in a while." Mom turned the heat under her frying pans to low and walked over to Dad's side.

"Matthew, why don't you go out and help your dad. When you strong boys are done, we can all have breakfast and then gather the Easter eggs!" Her fingers wiggled through my hair like racing worms.

Gripping his hands with mine, the scabs and scars of his workman's skin rough against my indolent flesh, Dad became a paternal pulley, leaning farther and farther back, bending his knees to gain enough leverage to get my nearly five hundred pounds off the sofa. After smoothing out the deep creases in the cushions where my body, the asteroid, had cratered the surface, I followed him through the kitchen and out the back door.

Dad's crab-grass infested front lawn, although typically manicured, had reeked of feces for at least five years. After the sewer's main line refused to digest one more feminine hygiene product, the oak tree's roots attacked its narrow passages with an army of sliver-thin growths. A pool of waste settled four inches from the front sidewalk and, despite Dad's efforts, could not be stopped unless we dug up the old septic tank and replaced it with a new one.

We constructed a makeshift bridge of plywood to cover the cesspool and keep my three-year-old niece Chelsey from accidentally falling into the foul, bubbling waste while collecting her Easter eggs. Carrying the wood a hundred feet from the garage to the front sidewalk had raised my heart rate, and sweat coated my underarms, inner thighs, and stomach. It all seemed like too much work to me, even if there was candy at the end of this rainbow.

"If I step on the board, will I fall through?" I asked as I dangled my mammoth sneakers over the corner. Shoe to wood, I anchored my foot into the cover and pushed down. Black liquid bubbled out from underneath each corner, and my leg began to surf across the soupy ground.

"You shouldn't. It's pretty strong stuff," Dad said, brushing away the wood shavings that clung like feeding ticks to his sweatshirt.

"What if I jump on it?"

"Matthew, why would you want to jump on a pile of crap?"

"Just because," I whimpered, tempting the situation by once again placing my foot on the board. "Why, am I too heavy for it to support?"

"No one should jump on this thing unless they are prepared to be knee-deep in stink."

He's avoiding my question, I thought, *because I'm too fat to stand here and he's too nice to tell the truth.*

The front door whipped open as we walked back toward the garage, striking the rust-pimpled siding with a crack.

"Uncle Matty! Grandpa! Look at all of the Easter eggs!" Chelsey was streaking across the front porch in her purple dinosaur pajamas, her arms bursting open like a flower on fast-forward. Bending at the waist, I opened my arms to meet her, hoisting her sleight body off of the ground and into my arms.

"Chelsey, how many Easter eggs do you think there are out there?"

"At least a hundred!"

"I'll bet that the Easter Bunny saw you helping Grandma with the dishes last night and decided you deserved all of the eggs he could get his paws on. I'll bet there are a million eggs in the front yard alone!" My thick fingers brushed the blond curls from her penetrating blue eyes. I couldn't remember being that small.

Chelsey leapt out of my arms, grabbed my wrist, and took off at a sprint. Her miniature hand guided me from tree to tree, from the mailbox to the clay flowerpot by the front door, as we sprinted after eggs. Sweat beads dripped from my forehead into my eyes. As we rounded the garden adjacent to the back porch, my breath turned shallow and my heartbeat thudded in my chest, neck, and head.

"Come on, Matty, let's go!" Running through water would have been easier than forcing my fat thighs, pressed and sticking together, to churn through the overgrown grass.

Colored eggs began to twist into kaleidoscopes as the thumping in my temples amplified. Chelsey's hand, dampened by my sweat, slipped from my grasp. Flashing lights from her sneaker heels blinked in front of me, her thin yellow hair flying like a trail of dust; I was losing her with each step. I couldn't catch my breath: it seized in my throat like a tightening noose, and the armpits, back, and stomach of my oversize T-shirt were soaked with perspiration.

I am having a heart attack, I thought. Bent over at the waist, my stomach cramped slightly and vomit burned in my esophagus. *I am going to die at sixteen.*

"Uncle Matty, look at all of my eggs!" Chelsey lifted the overflowing basket into the air and waved it, as if weightless, in her arms. All of the weight, it seemed, was on me. Labored, heavy breaths that burned my lungs with cold air began to subside as I watched my favorite person lower her basket and skip toward an egg tucked inside the lid of the propane tank. April's cool breeze struck my cheek with a gentle smack, and with a hitherto unknown clarity, I understood for the first time that my niece with the fat uncle would be my niece with no uncle in a matter of fifteen years or less.

Bags of potato chips, cartons of Little Debbie snack cakes, and the late-night leftover binges that calmed my anxiety on nights I felt alone would send me to my velvet-lined casket before she graduated high school.

"I'm going to miss it all," I said out loud, my eyes blurry from panicked tears that mixed with the sweat dripping from my forehead and rolled into my reddened eyes. "I'm never going to see her grow up and I'm never going to have kids of my own. I'm dying."

Chelsey ran up to me and grabbed my hand, placing her basket next to my size-sixteen feet. "Matty, are you okay? Don't you want to find eggs with me anymore?"

Before I had a chance to elaborate, to tell her that I loved her and would do whatever it took to be there for her life, the backdoor opened and Mom stepped out onto the splintered deck. She was now fully clothed in blue cotton stretch pants and a white sweatshirt with an appliqué bunny. Twirling her hands in half circles, like a kindergarten teacher rounding up her class after recess, she shouted, "Come on in—it's time for breakfast! We've got to get eatin' and on the road by eleven so we can get to Aunt Rosie's by lunchtime."

Chelsey picked up her basket and ran toward the house, but I couldn't move my feet. Either life or death had sent me a warning that if I stayed the course I would be doing far more of the latter than the former, and the message turned me into a modern-day Atlas. Five minutes passed and I had yet to move an aching muscle. As my heart rate slowed and my sweating receded to a trickle, it was no longer physical anguish that kept me fixed to the ground. I was scared of going inside the home that had, up to this point, been the epicenter of my indulgences. Mom yelled one more time, but I couldn't decipher a word she said. I simply walked toward the house, toward the sound of her voice, allowing my instincts to chart my path.

Later, at breakfast, I skipped the eggs, bacon, pancakes, and sausages, and instead made myself one slice of unbuttered toast. Toast would keep me alive for Chelsey, and for my own children, who's innocence would resurrect me again, just like my niece did on the day she saved my life and reminded me that more than anything, I wanted a Chelsey of my own someday.

Chapter 8

. . . .

Faults, Fertility Fears, and Testicles on Ice

Constance and I committed to having sex both early and often, waking daily before the sun crashed into the snow in order to crash into each other. Day after day, the programmed coffee maker infused our veiled bedroom with robust French aromas, an aphrodisiac for the early riser, and the alarm clock rang like a signal to the start of a race with no conceivable end.

We invested our mornings in sex on a mission that yielded nothing more than four darkened eyelids, two aggravated downstairs neighbors, and one negative pregnancy test.

Running my fingers along her stark white spine, skating my knuckles in imperfect figure eights from the base of her back to the nape of her neck, and burying my nose in her lavender-scented curls, our birth-control–free lovemaking remained as passionate and carefree as our days of pleasure-only intercourse.

Carrot, Ramona, and Cleo continued to perch above our heads as unyielding feline spectators, the honey-colored wood bed frame continued to creak at every toss or turn and the faux rotary phone continued, without fail, to rattle the bed-side table until the inquisitive tidings of one of our parents echoed from the answering machine down the hall. Nothing had changed except the possibility of a baby. We even adopted a puppy, Marcy, the half beagle, and convinced ourselves it wasn't a canine stand-in for the baby that wouldn't come.

During the first six months of attempted conception without successful commingling of egg and sperm, we never once pointed a finger at Constance's ovaries or my testicles in the literal or figurative sense. Somewhere around the close of month six, however, our disappointment divided the sum of our sexual experiences into one part physical pleasure and one part armchair science.

Constance's e-mails to me began to shift from the singularly coy and covert flirtations of a devoted lover to the inquisitions and not-so-subtle information sharing of a mild hypochondriac. My wife quickly developed a habit of loading my work inbox with studies celebrating the quality and quantity of predawn semen, and upon the occasion that six such messages appeared in under an hour, I realized that the heretofore absent, blaming finger was beginning its ascension in my general direction.

With or without spoken words, blaming digits, or understated e-mails, though, my self-suspicion had been mounting, and I was more than a little certain that the culprits behind our unpregnant state resided in my trousers.

"Baby, I have to be honest with you: I just know this is all my doing," I wrote to Constance in response to yet another email titled SIMPLE AND EFFECTIVE METHODS TO INCREASE YOUR CHANCES OF GETTING PREGNANT, which I determined, after sorting through my "Personal" e-mail folder, was a repeat offender from the prior week. "I just know the reason we don't have a baby on the way is because I used to be a big fat fattie. You know how I am. I'm constantly worried about what the long-term ramifications of having been five hundred pounds will be. I've always been nervous my heart would one day explode like a cupcake hit by a Hummer, but now I'm starting to get the feeling that all of those years of entrapment and friction have turned my fellas against me. Why doth my reproductives hate me so?"

An hour of e-mail silence ticked by, and with my egregiously large coffee standing on its final quivering legs, there was nothing to support me except the spotty glass desktop covered with printouts of the syndicated fitness articles I had printed for my portfolio. I laid my head on the glass and gazed at my shoes through the pane, wondering if my mammoth feet would look odd when juxtaposed on a child that could sprout anywhere between Constance's diminutive five-two frame and my six-four stature. I pressed my head harder into the desk, applying sufficient pressure to impress my skin and smudge the glass further with facial oil. Visions of a baby with Constance's adorable face and my freakishly large shoes repulsed me, and I prayed to nothing in particular that our child wouldn't be burdened with disproportionately large feet.

I want to be able to put my baby's whole foot into my mouth someday, I thought as the chime of incoming e-mails struck an audible chord resonating from my ears straight to my quickened heartbeat.

Constance had written back to deflect my digital claim with a profession of love and a written nod to my "beautiful face." Leaving no thread hanging, she promised we'd talk about it later over a bowl of steaming butternut squash soup. On the occasion that my physical attributes enter any given conversation as a means of abating tension, it's akin to throwing a watermelon on a trampoline and waiting for the inevitable explosion—my conjecture was as good as gravity. "And by the way, have I told you lately how much I loathe Hummers?" she wrote in closing. "How dare you put them in the same sentence with something as brilliant as cupcakes."

The giant forehead smudge clinging to my desk was too distracting to work through, so I grabbed the Windex from my boss's file cabinet and wiped away the memory of my would-be-baby's grotesquely giant foot.

I felt like the hypothetical Hummer had already turned me, the cupcake, into a scattering of crumbs.

"I don't want to be insistent about something for which I have zero substantiated proof," I said later that night over my steaming bowl of soup that was as much a beauty treatment as it was a means of sustenance. "But I know obesity is a major factor in infertility because the genitals get overheated and the sperms die. Hot sperms are unhappy sperms."

Soup had become our main source of sustenance after Constance read a book about the French paradox of thinness, and it took very little time for me to rely on the vegetable-based heat that billowed into my face to dissipate my post-work haze.

"But you haven't been overweight for almost ten years," Constance said, "and your sperms have had more than enough time to rejuvenate. I think you're giving them way more credit than they deserve." Her ripe blue eyes danced with an unfair advantage usually reserved for adoptable puppies in a box; the owners of which were clever enough to know that all adorable things are made even more so when placed inside of a box. Constance's box, however, was closing in around me.

"But maybe my extreme fatness unleashed some sort of semen genocide, wiped me out completely, and now there's nothing left to carry on," I said.

"That's just stupid, Matty. I think we should give it a few months of having sex early in the morning during our fertile period, and then we'll go from there."

After twenty-eight weeks with only one late period—the mysterious ten-day anomaly—it didn't seem so much stupid as it did an unfortunate product of reality. I couldn't stop focusing on my depleted army of sperm and the nagging suspicion that the extra skin at the tops of my legs was unwittingly wiping out my troops. Average, virile young men focus brain cells on ESPN and figuring out how to turn any leftover food into an innovative burrito—not sperm counts. However, because of my prior obesity, I privately had been ceding gray matter to the concern for several years.

Constance was not about to budge, so I quietly finished my soup and agreed to give it another two months. Shortly thereafter, we headed out for our nightly walk through Winnemac Park, which, like the soup, was also an import from France. *Perhaps,* I thought, *we should contact the French embassy to inquire if they have any paradoxes focusing on conception.*

"Damn it!" Constance yelled from the bathroom, slamming something I could hear against something I couldn't see. Without leaving my red-pepper frittata unattended on the stove to follow her cry, and without a verbal inquiry into the nature of her expletive, I knew that a Sunday night bathroom break had morphed into a harbinger of bad news.

Our baby was currently not growing inside Constance.

I wanted to ask the question someone in love is supposed to instinctively ask—"Are you okay?"—and I wanted to run to her side and hold her while she cried on the toilet and tell her that this was just another month I'd get to have her all to myself. And I did exactly that, but it took me a minute to unglue my eyes from the frittata, which had begun to bubble and burn in the bottom of the Wok.

Nine months and nine menstrual cycles had now passed, and upon the arrival of blood, we knew that morning intercourse could no longer be deemed a fail-safe solution for our inability to conceive.

"Well, I guess we officially have a problem," Constance said.

"Yes," I replied as I took the tear-stained toilet paper from her hands, rolled it into a ball, and threw it down the hallway. Flashes of fur whizzed past the door as three cats pursued the makeshift toy. "Now it's business."

Constance scoured the Internet the following day, and we mutually agreed over e-mail it was time to edit all of the fun from our existence because, according to the experts, there was simply no other way to make a baby. My obese childhood, however, was still not part of the explanation.

Over dinner that night, fanned across our dining-room table were stacks of literature from every nook of the natal industry that proffered how vital it is for a man to have sex in the early morning if conception is problematic. That simplistic and rather harmless advice, which some doctors purport has no bearing on conception, was also accompanied by an evil litany of off-limits activities on which Cleo the cat had curled into a purring ball. Before sinking into slumber, as she clawed and dug at the papers, Cleo just as easily could have turned the bad news bearers into a litter box, but unaware that the words beneath her were a silencing decree for her owners, she instead went the route of any self-respecting cat and licked herself into a coma.

No hot baths, no long periods of sitting, no alcohol, no long-distance running, no masturbation, and no tight under-wear, the latter having not been a factor since the first month of our relationship when Constance politely urged me to make the switch to boxer briefs.

"I really shouldn't be having wine anyway," Constance said, dragging her fork like a dagger through a pile of polenta before taking a sip of Petite Syrah and stabbing me through the heart. "It's not good for women when they're trying to conceive, and even though we only have it a couple of times a week, I think we should stop altogether."

I snatched my glass and poured the peppery blend over my lips, past my gums, and stood witness as my favorite morning activities were about to disappear as quickly as what stood to be my final glass of wine. Many of them I delivered to the executioner on my own accord, betraying myself in the name of bettering my "self," beginning with my favorite nonsexual activity.

"I know I workout too hard, so I'll cut back my mileage to twenty-five a week," I said as I mentally packed on ten pounds upon said agreement to become a less-active man. "That should help keep my body temperature lower."

Eight miles per day, five days per week, and zero children wasn't a winning equation. In spite of my running addiction, my need to slam my feet onto the pavement to escape a past that was constantly breathing down my neck, I was willing to excise mileage for the good of our tireless reproductive journey.

"Yeah, you know on the days you workout, you're always really hot for the whole day after that, 'cuz your metabolism is so high," Constance said. "And like we've talked about before, I really think you need to eat more. I mean, you're six-four and you eat as much as me. That's not right."

I pressed my forehead into my palms and began to grind, mortar-and-pestle style, the sharp pain blooming in my frontal lobe until it was reduced to a skittering throb. Extreme to extreme, I had swung from the basement of health to the pitch of the roof, and my selective diet housed very little room for upward expansion. Few ideas terrified me more than the prospect of increasing the amount of food I ate each day.

Most days I burned more calories than I consumed and burned just as much energy obsessing about the nutrients that had passed my lips. Losing the weight, shedding myself of the pounds upon pounds that were capable of ending my life by age thirty did not rid me of the feeling that I was an out-of-control eater. We agreed, however, that I could, without weight gain, stand to up my intake of natural fats like nuts, avocados, and olive oil. A switch to two-percent milk was my final concession.

Small budges to begin with will get us our baby, I thought.

We also agreed that I would begin perching myself on the front edge of my office chair to allow my testicles ample breathing space during eight hours of sedentary office work. If that didn't suffice, Constance urged me to substitute my standard variety chair with a yoga ball—a woman at her office did it to aid an ailing back. Knowing full well I'd never take a yoga ball to work in the instance of a bad back or a hot body, I agreed.

And finally, without broaching the topic candidly, we decided that my only moments of intimate pleasure would occur with Constance in the room.

"You know, I guess we'll just have to save up your stuff and have sex every other day to up our chances," Constance said in perhaps the sweetest, least direct delivery of the "stop-masturbating" decree any husband has ever received. Masturbation is not a topic we are too prudish to confront at the dinner table, but that night it felt parental and icky. I knew she was right, and I again acquiesced to her suggestion not because the most wonderful woman in the world asked me to do so and not because I thought it would actually get us pregnant, but because I was convinced my sperm count was low, and none of these solutions were as embarrassing or harrowing as going to the doctor to find out my stuff was bad.

As I swished the last ounce of wine between my teeth, forcing the grainy sediment through the gaps of my crooked smile, I was overcome with an urge to divulge a secret I had been keeping for weeks. With nothing but the dregs of polenta and wine left between us, Constance had unabashedly set the record straight about the changes I needed to make in my life to make this baby a reality. I figured I owed it to her bravery to summon a little courage of my own.

"Oh, and there's one other thing I read about online that helps, especially for people with high body temperatures," I said, constricting my throat in order to scrape any remaining essence of wine from my esophagus. Courage via vino, courtesy of the five years of on-again, off-again wine-appreciation lessons I'd received in drunken doses from Richard, my father-in-law.

I lowered my head and voice, a drawbridge reluctantly inviting foot traffic to proceed with caution across barracuda-infested waters. "I read that men with high body temperatures should ice themselves regularly," I said.

"You mean, ice yourself . . . down there?" Constance asked, pressing her thighs together and pointing her finger toward her lap, a charade signifying the potential unification of ice and genitalia.

"Apparently applying ice packs to your testicles creates an environment conducive to sperm production," I said. "One hour a day while your legs are elevated provides the best results."

"That makes sense, I guess," she said. "Are you going to do it?"

"Yes, I'm going to do it. I mean, if it helps, if putting ice on my balls really works, then it's worth it."

"Are you okay?" Constance asked as she dragged the edge of her hand along my bare torso, stopping above my navel to write "I love you" with her index finger. My feet, elevated by a stack of throw pillows cushioning the backs of my knees, were blocking the bottom of the TV at the foot of our bed.

"I love you," I said, emphasizing the *you* to let her know I had received her hand-written message. Constance flattened her palm on my stomach and swiped it back and forth, erasing the imaginary words from my body.

"Does it hurt?" she asked.

"Yes, it hurts," I said. "I just want to lie here and watch episodes of *Arrested Development* until my hour is up because that will keep me from thinking about exactly how much this sucks."

"We need to have sex tonight, though," Constance said, reaching beneath the sheets toward my frozen midsection. "Is now an okay time to touch you, to get started?"

Three weeks into icing and the mild-mannered, indie

music lover that once lived in my home and inhabited my body with a smile on his face and a song burgeoning from his lips had turned into an epic, Hans Christian Anderson—era bitch. A question like "Is now an okay time to touch you?" would have been redundant and irrelevant. Testosterone was now filling me in ways I had never experienced, and when I wasn't livid as a result of every minor hiccup in my life that would have normally slid off my untroubled back, I was ready to ravage my wife at any turn.

When the surges waned, however, and my hormones evened out, I found myself staring at the same *Rolling Stone* album review for forty minutes straight and feeling impossibly sad and disappointed that I had managed to squander my musical talent before the age of thirty, while Avril Lavigne lived to score a second hit record. I flooded Avril's glam, immature face with my tears, and sealed my eyes for a nap.

～

"I can't even think straight anymore," I told my lifelong friend Mary over lunch at Spacca Napoli, an authentic pizzeria one block from my office. "I'm always ready to nap, I stare at my work and try to read these stories I have to edit, and I end up stuck on the same paragraph for twelve consecutive reads. My brain cramps whenever I try to make a decision, and I get tears in my eyes every time someone doesn't give me the exact support or reaction I'm expecting. I don't want to talk or be talked to, and I don't want to be touched. Constance's words are so sweet, and she's trying so hard to be supportive, but my mind is in constant combat mode, and I can't help but find fault in everything she says or does. And then, after we fight, I want to have crazy animal sex. It's not me, and I feel poisoned and sick."

Mary's laugh echoed in the brick and tile room, and she covered her mouth with the cloth napkin to prevent buffalo mozzarella from flying onto the patrons next to us, who were casting riled glances in our direction. An intimate and boisterous discussion of my testicles was not kosher material for the Ravenswood Avenue lunch crowd. Reproductive health was not a part of their lunchtime plan, but like most realities, plans are futile.

"Boy, you've just suffered through four weeks of nasty-ass PMS," Mary said. "I mean, it's like the same thing really, don't you think? I can see it, behind your eyes, there's a caveman peering out, ready to beat his chest and defend his woman. Icing has unleashed your beast, and now you're like one of those hypermasculine frat boys who listens to the Dave Matthews Band and has a constant erection."

An actress and writer of considerable talent, Mary has a honed knack for turning the tumultuous into living theater. Sitting in my hand-carved chair, licking the pizza sauce off the back of my wrist, I listened as Mary rewrote my past month as a sitcom that toted the line between risqué, tragic, and juvenile.

"That's not me, Mary."

"Well, baby, it just might be until you get pregnant, so you should consider heading to Boy's Town, investing in a loincloth, and having some fun with it. Manly men are sexy, too, you know."

I chuckled in spite of my new masculine self because I knew she was insightful for having pinned me as the latest caveman in a world teeming with cavemen. And it was worth a laugh, but it was a deplorable epiphany nonetheless that the sensitive feminist I'd carefully crafted myself to be could so easily get uprooted by a daily ice pack between my thighs.

Then two days after my lunch with Mary two days after I was outed as a manly man—Constance got her period for the tenth month in a row, and I stood in the bathroom over a bloody letdown, never having felt like less of a man in my entire life.

"I think it's time," I said. "We should just spend the money and buy an over-the-counter sperm test so I can know it's my fault already."

"It's not about finding fault," Constance said as she reached up to stroke my forearm.

"It's easy to say that when you're not the one to blame, and you're not the one who has to ice his genitals every night," I cried. "I just want to know for sure that it's my fault, and then we can move on to something that's actually going to work for us. I just need to know."

One trip to the pharmacy, two home-fertility tests, and four days later, I officially had a low sperm count, and our inability to conceive finally attached itself to the word we had avoided uttering in ten months of unsuccessful sex.

We were infertile, and it was, indeed, my fault.

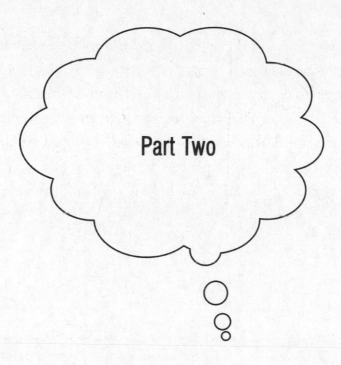

Part Two

So This Sperm Walks
into a Lab . . .

Chapter 9

. . . .

Dr. GQ, Walling Babies, and the Bathroom of Sin

The only urology office sanctioned by our insurance company was on the top floor in the last room lining the solitary, half-lit hallway at Swedish Covenant Hospital. After urology, there was no more hospital of which to speak, a sadistic metaphor for the future of the patients who were banished to the bowels of the medical world.

First comes incontinence, then comes death.

It was a full house that day; just me and the saddest, most burdened group of late-life men waiting for the urinary yeomen to guide us through the gates of emasculated hell. Odors akin to nutmeg and spoiled milk tainted the air, and with each breath, with each glance lingering too long at the purplish leathery skin of the man next to me, I became acutely aware that I was supposed to be riddled with shame just for being there.

"Tucking a urology office in the outermost reaches of a hospital where the only restroom is more than twenty exam rooms away?" I said to Constance in a low, but not low enough voice. "I mean, really? I perish to think of the emergencies that have arisen for my geriatric brethren, shuffling around with walkers and battling bladders that have long since lost their youthful control." Based on hospital positioning alone, the male urinary and reproductive systems appeared to be the most shameful in the Land of Oz.

When my name was called, I felt guilty for not letting everyone else go first. I had a lot of life left to live, I hoped, and waiting a few more hours for my turn would have been a respectful gift. It also would have been the perfect time killer. *Shy* is not a word often used in conjunction with my name, but knowing I was about to go in and drop my pants in front of a complete stranger, one who would inevitably stick his finger up my butt, didn't even justify my work-free afternoon.

"I hope he's ugly and old," I said to Constance, knowing full well that urologists, proctologists, and gynecologists are without fail the most attractive group of specialists in the medical industry.

"I'm sure he'll be a cute little old guy, like my dad," Constance said.

"Please, never again mention your dad as I'm about to get my goods checked out," I said. I hung up my coat, scarf, and bag on the back of the exam room door and then began to fish around my bag for the camera. "Let's take some pictures to remember this day."

Picture number one was a candid photo, our signature pose, with the camera held at arm's length to capture our smiling faces on our first urological vacation. It would earn a place in the photo album alongside other great adventures, from London to Dublin to Disneyland to urologist. As I snapped the first photo, the flash forced a brilliant light into our eyes just as the nurse opened the door, urine sample cup in hand.

"Sir, I'm going to need a urine sample from you. Do you think you can go?" she asked with a valley-girl intonation, her eyes bugging out as if she had a sudden onset of a thyroid condition.

"I can always go," I said, handing the camera to Constance and following the nurse out the door. Nurse Befuddled handed me the pee cup, her head shaking back and forth like the slight, constant corrections of a steering wheel in the hands of an actor pretending to drive. It was obvious that not every urology visit doubled as a photo op.

After I gave her what she came for and returned to the exam room, I proceeded to pose with a plastic model of the four sections of the bladder. Next I held aloft a model of the inner workings of the male reproductive system. Each plastic model was lifted from the table and propped next to my face. I contorted my expressions from confusion to surprise to disgust as Constance snapped shot after shot. Feeling frisky in an unexpected venue, I played up my first photo shoot, giving each take my all. Flashing lights and make believe distracted me from what was to become reality in less than two minutes.

"These will be great for your blog," Constance said. "Pictures from the penis front." Blogging was something I had thought about doing for the health-and-wellness website I run, but initially I had imagined blogging about weight loss. My boss, Mary Connors, once told me that readers like to read the words and stories of people who are actually going through something. And since I knew I'd have to tell her about our troubles at some point, I decided that what I was going through was worth writing about.

One knock-knock was a call to action as the door opened to reveal, as expected, a thirty-something male with perfectly coiffed hair, intimidating white straight teeth, and the kind of bone structure only doctors on television are legally allowed to have. I immediately felt fat and ugly, and the crookedness of my teeth seemed less quirky than British.

"Hi, I'm Dr. GQ," he said as he pushed his clammy hand into my rigid fist. "So tell me why you're here."

Silence. Silence. Barriers were erected in my mind to avoid thinking about Mr. Popular, former high-school quarterback, king of the prom staring at my probably-smaller-than-his penis, judging the unexplained scars and sagging skin on my imperfect, formerly fat body. Nothing I could conjure could stop me from believing that Dr. GQ, top in his class and first in the hearts of women everywhere, was feasting on the short-comings of the most masculine area of my body where no such failings existed for him. His sharpest worry was ensuring that his two point five children got into the best Chicago academy and buffing his Jaguar convertible until it shined so purely he could stare longingly into the paint job as if it were a one-hundred-thousand dollar mirror. A reflection of his perfect life.

Constance, an angel sans wings, granted my prayers and broke the iceberg with a verbal mallet. "Well, we've been trying to conceive for ten months," she said, "but to no avail."

"We just thought I should get everything checked out," I stammered, coughing to loosen the words from my throat. I took a deep breath and exhaled—a cooling teakettle—allowing my breath to pass through my lips with an audible wisp. "I just thought it would be best to make sure my sperm count was okay."

We took turns telling him about the intricacies of our reproductive failings and reiterating that our goals for this exam were to get a fuller picture of our reproductive situation.

"I mean, I'm not hoping I have a low count," I said, "but I'm just hopeful we can avoid sending Constance in for more invasive excavations, if you know what I mean."

Dr. GQ laughed—not too loud and not too soft, not too nasally and not too throaty—and ran his fingers through mounds of George Clooney hair, at which time I was almost certain he nodded at my bald scalp and gave me an exaggerated, all-knowing wink. A wink that whispered in tones heard only by the bald, *Sorry about the hair loss, Mr. Clean. I've got eight strands sprouting out of every follicle on my head.*

"First things first; I'm going to give you a full exam," he said. "Make sure you don't have any kinks or blockages. Then I'll send you down to the lab for some blood tests and a semen analysis. With the analysis, you'll have to do two of them, one today and one three days from now. Sperm counts change from day to day, so to get a full picture, we need to do two."

In what was becoming one of my least suave encounters with another human being, I cocked my head to the left side and blinked at Dr. GQ. And then I blinked again, saying nothing in response to the litany of orders he outlined.

"Okay then," he said. "I guess we need to get started. Just go ahead and take down your pants and we'll get going. It's up to you if you want your wife to stay."

"She can stay," I said with a quasi-shout, trying to prove through volume and decisiveness that I had nothing to hide and no shame clinging to my sexuality, no leach intent on draining me of my pride. Dr. GQ be damned, I was a virile man. I unbuttoned my pants and in one fell swoop forced my jeans and underwear into a pool around my ankles. His gloved hands dug into my testicles, twisting them from side to side before he pushed his finger underneath the sac at the very top and began squeezing the skin.

"I'm looking for any sort of kink or enlarged vein that could be blocking things," he said. "But everything feels great so far."

Damn right it's great, I thought, because as much as I

wanted a solution, I didn't want to know my manhood had failed—that my manhood was somehow lesser than those of the skinny, fit men I had spent my adolescence loathing.

"Now I'm going to need to check your prostate," he said. If words are indeed like weapons, his were a machete to my tightened throat. Being a man not averse to all things anal, I still had a sad spot in my heart for the rough rectal exam. One finger covered in lube, a poke and a prod done rapidly and without finesse, it underscored the lack of understanding most men have regarding how to treat a hole. "Do you want your wife to step out now?"

"Sure," I said. Vulnerable as I had been standing naked, having my junk prodded by a stranger, for Constance to stand witness as I bent over the lab table would have left nothing of me for only me. Constance grabbed her coat and patted me on the shoulder as she passed between Dr. GQ and me. Stiff hinges slowly coerced the door from its wide-open stance to a distancing crack. I cheered for a catch as the light from the hallway faded and the latch clicked, sending my butt muscles into an involuntarily clench.

Turn around, bend over, and groan. When it's all done, be silent and pretend nothing just happened.

"Well, everything from the exam seems fine," Dr. GQ said. There's no swelling of the prostate, which is a very good thing. Why don't you go ahead and pull your pants back up and meet me at the front desk for a deposit cup and a lab order."

I collected the two lab orders and began the long walk back to the elevator bank. Constance and I went down to the first floor, registered at the desk, and then sat in the waiting area for my name to be called.

"How are you doing?" she asked as she stroked my forearm. Three shrieking kids ran circles around a coffee table filled with sections of the *Chicago Tribune*, one child holding a Dora the Explorer doll and trying to keep the others from placing their hands on her felt face. Two women in burkas sat to our left and whispered quietly in words I didn't understand. Four babies held in the arms of their mothers fell like dominoes, one by one, into fevered wails. Two nurses stationed behind the counter were chatting about how much weight they both had put on over the holidays and how impossible it has been, two months later, to come to terms with their new sizes.

I wasn't doing well. Dr. GQ handed me a plastic cup and sent me on my way, and never once did Pretty Boy, M.D., put into words what I reluctantly figured out for myself. My semen sample was going to be done right there, right then, in the lab of the hospital. George Michael, Pee Wee Herman, Matt Miller—masturbating in public was forced onto my docket, and unlike those publicly lewd celebrities, I wasn't given a choice.

"This sucks," I said. "I don't even know what to expect at this point. I definitely didn't expect to have a wank at the hospital. Will there be magazines and stuff in a quiet room where I just go and do my business? I mean, that's how it's done in movies and on TV."

"It's gotta be something like that," Constance said. "I wish I could go with you and give you a hand."

Trepidation was no match for my desire, and her words began a familiar tingle in my groin. "Yeah, well, something tells me the nurses aren't going to be so keen on the idea of you coming in with me," I said.

"Plus it would be kind of weird," she said. "Having everybody know what you're doing."

"Yeah, tell me about it," I said. Locked doors are no barrier for a stigma so powerful some believe it to be a blindness-inducing sin. If Jesus didn't want you to masturbate, he certainly didn't want you to do it in a public gathering spot dedicated to healing. Healing would have nothing to do with my dirty little not-so secret. Never did I think that something so rote, a right of pleasure passage so natural and calming, could become dreadful with one undecipherable scribble of a doctor's pen.

"Matthew Miller?"

My name echoed throughout the waiting room, floating like a question with no answer, or at least an answer I didn't want to provide. An answer that would lead me to an undisclosed masturbatorium where all the nurses would know exactly what I was up to.

One kiss on the lips from Constance gave me the nerve to

force my feet onto the Berber carpeting, stand erect, and walk toward Nurse Awkward.

"Hello, Mr. Miller. How are you today?" she asked.

"Good," I lied, unwilling to give her the satisfaction of knowing that I was teeth-grindingly nervous about the moment at hand.

"All right, so you'll first want to wash your hands before depositing the sample in that cup," she said. "When you're done, twist the lid until you hear a click. That means it's locked. Then just put it in the little door in the wall and let me know when you're done."

"Oh, so, I'm going to be doing this, here?" I asked. "In the bathroom?"

"Yep," she said, smoothing the frizzy black hairs that were popping out of the top of her ponytail. Nurse Awkward began walking back to her station, stopped in her tracks, and then, as if mimicking a shampoo commercial, threw her head back over her shoulder. "Don't forget to let me know when you're finished."

No magazines, no videos, no comfy chair, no lab table to prop myself on, just one dingy, single-person public restroom, a mirror, and a lurking nurse waiting for me to finish masturbating so the next normal urine-sample patient could take my place. Behind my thin door, I could hear poked and prodded babies screaming, high-heeled shoes clacking like urgent type-writers up and down the hallway, nurses and patients chatting about the unseasonably warm weather, and I stood with my pants gathered around my ankles for the second time in twenty minutes.

Arousal minus mental stimulation was one obstacle; another was duration. As much as I wanted to start pulling and get it over with, I also wanted to make sure I didn't finish too quickly. Walking up to the nurse five minutes later would seem too rushed, as if I had been only too eager to do what I was about to do. But I also didn't want to linger and make her think I was lost in the moment, enjoying the freedom of permitted public release. Ten minutes would do, I decided, and began the long road down my sample-producing journey.

Only five minutes later, not a creature was stirring and no amount of caressing or imaginary scenarios involving me, Constance, and a bowl of bananas Foster could move the needle closer to solid. I opened my eyes and stared at myself in the mirror. Dark circles stormed beneath my eyelids and the overhead fluorescents were unkind to my depleted hairline, which was in need of a shave.

"What is wrong with you?" I asked myself, watching my dry lips open and close. My crooked teeth looked overwhelmingly askew. "You can and have done this in your sleep. Just pull yourself together already and make it happen." I closed my eyes once again and bid farewell to the ugly image from the mirror. Fluorescent lights made me look pale and aged, and with my pants around my ankles, I had never felt less attractive or more pathetic.

I sucked four deep breaths in and out of my gut, breaths that with each exhale sent mental versions of screaming babies, nurses, the unfinished book in my bag, and the unfortunate reflection of my sailing off on the strings of green balloons. Balloon therapy was a trick I'd learned from my therapist in Minneapolis back when I suffered from postcollege, I-can't-believe-I'm-working-retail anxiety. Now that I had overcome said anxiety, and the embarrassment of conjuring rubber balloons to soothe my soul had waned, it remained the singular weapon I had on deck to right the ship.

Five minutes later, I placed my sample in the wall box and entered the hallway to inform the nurse I had finished. Ten minutes later I was at home, in bed, with a pint of vanilla ice cream and a demand for silence. I fell asleep with a spoon in my hand and didn't wake up until the smell of pasta and pancetta poked my nose.

"Thank you for doing this," Constance said, pushing the half-empty bottle of Mark West pinot noir directly between us. That night we decided we could risk our temporary fertility health for the sake of some spiritual wine. Masturbating in public was reason enough to forget the baby and remember the drink. "You know, a lot of guys wouldn't be so eager to find out about their sperm counts."

"I can see why," I said.

"You know what I mean," she said. "I appreciate you taking such good care of us and our family. It means a lot to me that you're willing to do whatever it takes to figure this out. I want you to know that I'm proud of you, and that I'll do the same if we need to."

"Thank you," I said. It was less than seventy-two hours until I had to do it all over again, and I still knew that this was all my fault.

❦

Phone calls with my parents often skirted the topic of where we were in the reproduction process. Not once follow ing an around-the-horn update of the entire Miller team or a local weather report did I find an opening to insert my pro-jected sperm-count issue. Mom and Dad, I knew, did not want to be intrusive, but the issue itself was leprosy, and I was the infected limb dancing circles around their half-horrified, half-repulsed faces.

"So, I just wanted to let you know that I've been going to the doctor to make sure my sperm count is okay," I said. I told them about the negative home tests and my disturbing moments of solitude performing solo along to a canned sound-track of babies and high heels blaring in the background.

"I'll bet you made sure that door was locked nice and

tight," Dad said, laughing, his labored breath a bass drum pounding against the receiver.

"And be sure you hit the cup," Mom said, laughing in conjunction with Dad. "And don't overflow it like the first time you gave a urine sample."

Nobody had informed me when I was a child that a trace amount of urine was all that was required for testing. I learned this, via mocking laughter, after informing my mother and Aunt Dee during one of our trips to the Indianola clinic, "The cup was so full I almost spilled it putting it in the wall."

"I know it's kind of gross to hear about that, I'm sure," I said. "I mean, I won't make it a habit of telling you about my personal habits. But I just thought you might be curious about what's been going on."

"Hey, better you than me," my dad said. "You guys will get there. It just takes time."

"And it's nothing to be embarrassed about," Mom said. "You're just making sure everything's okay. I think that's a good thing. Just don't get too worried about it. I know sometimes that birth control just does horrible things, especially since Constance was on it for so long."

"Thanks," I said, skipping my chance to refute her medicinal curse as nothing more than wishful thinking. With the promise of calling them on Thursday after receiving the test results, we said our weekly good-byes.

Medicine did not stay in your system for ten months, and

the pharmacy dispenser of untaken pills that I had removed from the trash was simply not powerful enough to keep us childless from its rightful home in the medicine bin. Mom's wishful thinking was less wishful than a verbal plate of peanut-butter cookies baked to make me forget all about the problems at hand and fill the void with food. But I no longer found myself whole when the hole was merely patched with edible filler.

Pressing my nose against the red Oriental rug, my eyes sealed tight, I watched as Marcy, the puppy, Rachael Ray, ice packs, and my semen cup made their way into the atmosphere via imaginary balloons. On Saturday afternoon the balloons were black, likely because the Food Network was playing at a volume that exceeded my iced-testicle limits. One cold pack had been squeezed between my thighs for an hour, forcing my testicles up into my body and my body temperature to plummet.

"We should go soon," Constance said. "The lab is only open until four, and if there's a line, it could take a while."

"I have an idea," I said. "Let's not go. Instead we could stay home and reenact that one time when I was kidnapped by the Russian Mafia and forced to braid jump ropes filled with cocaine."

"What are you talking about?" Constance asked, lowering her home-decorating magazine, eyes squinted in parental-like confusion. "Are you having some sort of seizure from icing your balls?

"Never mind," I said. "Forget I said anything. Just give me five more minutes before you send me back to hell."

Not knowing what to expect was somehow easier than three full days disguised as a doomsday clock, and my current attitude moved Constance to the tipping point. Surliness was gasoline and I could not run without it. I could not make the fire burn any brighter, but Constance kept trying. She brought me Godiva truffles, massaged my shoulders, and partook of more tennis on television than any nonfanatic has a right to view. Yet regardless, I was irrational and selfish.

Fifty minutes later I pulled my size thirty-four jeans up around my hips, put my camouflage cardigan over my broad shoulders, and tightened the cap on the sample cup until, like a single cell of bubble wrap, it produced an audible snap. Producing the sample wasn't any easier the second time around. Mentally, it was more difficult to block out the babies and the nurses and the high-heel clacks, and the balloons to which I affixed my anxiety during the first go only sank to the ground this time.

It took fifteen minutes of pure speed action sans lotion or lubrication, solutions that would only taint the sample, to fulfill Dr. GQ's orders and lower the curtain on my days of hospital masturbation. When I opened the wall box to deposit my deposit, however, there were three other containers of undeterminable liquids inside. I merged my semen into the traffic jam of fluids and closed the door.

What if my sample gets switched? I thought. *I didn't come all this way to have my semen mixed up with another dude's spunk.* Careful, so as not to touch the cups that weren't products of my own body, I removed my semen from the wall and sat it on the ledge of the sink.

"Excuse me," I yelled across the hallway, my body wedged between the door and the jamb to keep the room and my sample invisible to passersby. "I went to put my sample in the wall, and there were already three other cups in there."

"Don't worry about it," the nurse said as she flicked her hand in front of her face as if pushing an unwanted fragrance out of her path. "Are your name and Social Security number on the cup?"

"Yes," I said. "But it seems kind of strange. I just don't want it to get mixed up."

"Sir, don't worry," she said. Her eyes had since drifted down to her clipboard to scan a list of things I knew nothing about. "Sometimes the lab gets backed up. I'll make sure they get them out of there right away."

Still baffled by the backup, I reentered the bathroom and returned my cup to the overfilled cabinet. Matthew M. F. Miller, followed by the nine digits of my identity, was imprinted on the caboose of the sample train. Nothing about it sat well with me. *All My Children* filled my childhood summer days, and I knew how little hospital staff could be trusted with the proper care of sperm. But I closed the door and left the hospital as fast as I could. I had three days before I found out that my sperm count was low, and I was going to make the most of it.

⌒⌒

The scene was the same—top-floor urology office—but the players had significantly changed. A lobby once filled to the brim with geriatric bladder cases was replaced with empty seats and one man in his late thirties reporting for his "procedure." Lack of clarity regarding the conversation between the man and the hospital staff regarding his "procedure" made me queasy. By their hushed tones and incomplete sentences, I concluded that he was about to undergo a life-saving bladderectomy. I felt great sadness for him on the cusp of losing his ability to pee on command, but it also made me feel better about the too-few-sperm message I was about to receive.

Constance had one of those important meetings with doughnuts, coffee, and spreadsheets, so I sat alone in the waiting room and flipped through the one magazine in the rack with Andre Agassi's face on the cover. Andre, father of two, eight-time Grand Slam tennis champion. Me, father failure and two-time hospital masturbator. Cover to cover, the entire magazine was devoted to living the good life, which according to the editors entailed consuming scads of rare Kobe beef, driving a sports car at illegal speeds, owning no fewer than four tailored Italian suits, and using your chiseled model-like face to win friends and influence people.

A good life, it appeared, was out of my reach due more to my inherently unmodel-like face than a lack of funds, which were a significant sticking point as well. Perhaps Constance and I could settle for the adequate life instead.

My first exam room would prove to be a rapid pit stop. "Can you give me a urine sample?" the nurse inquired.

"Always," I said. I can urinate on command, likely because I was constantly clutching a Starbucks cup or the water-filled glass that rarely got the opportunity to rest upon the top of my carafe.

When I finished and returned to the exam room, the nurse informed me that I'd be moving because a "procedure" was going to be taking place in my current room. She assured me that all patients would still be seen in order. I couldn't have cared less about that, but this mysterious "procedure" was starting to wear on my nerves.

Dr. GQ entered the second room before I even had a chance to hang my seven-foot Gap scarf on the peg.

"That's Gap, right? From, like, three years ago," he said.

"Yeah," I said, even though it was more like five years ago.

I expected more from him, from someone so obviously well-to-do, than tossing about knowledge and release dates of mass-market scarves that any struggling writer could own. Dr. GQ, perhaps, didn't adhere to the ascribed good life either.

"I've got the exact same one," he said as he pulled up the doctor-friendly wheelie chair. We finally had a bond, a rallying scarf that would personalize our relationship prior to the falling of the gauntlet about to chop off my masculinity. "Well, I have some good news. It looks like you're fine. Sperm counts are good. One was just slightly low, but counts change so much that we consider one test on the good side an okay result. One test was sixty million and one was ten, and we consider anything between twenty and eighty million an acceptable level. Your testosterone is also spot-on, and the two hormones in your brain that tell your testicles to make sperm are fine, too.

"So everything you've been doing, the icing, the vitamins, the reduced running, are all things you should be doing, and it seems to be working," he said. "My diagnosis is to go home right now, and give it a try. Go have some fun. That's the best part, right? The trying?"

"Definitely," I said. "That's the only good thing about all of this."

"What I really want you and your wife to do is give it three more months. Hit the reset button, start trying again, and if there's still nothing at that point, then she needs to get checked out. But you seem to be just fine. Just keep it fun. Stress can be a very bad thing in this process."

I thanked Dr. GQ, collected my coat and scarf, and began to don my winter costume.

"Have you seen any good movies lately?" he asked, opening the door and walking out into the hallway to place my blue chart in a bin marked COMPLETED.

"We just watched *The Departed* last night," I said. "It was really fun. And it didn't feel like a three-hour movie at all. I liked it a lot more than I thought I would."

"I've wanted to see that for so long," he said. "But we never get to the movies now that we've got a little one at home. Even DVDs over an hour and a half don't get watched. Being child-less is not such a bad thing. Enjoy your freedom while you have it."

Freedom is fluid, and I did not believe our inability to con-ceive somehow kept us free. Going to the movies on a Saturday afternoon and sleeping for eight consecutive hours were only two flavors of freedom, but these were the flavors that every parent seemed to scoop onto my dish whenever I bemoaned the fact that we couldn't get pregnant. Until we could not conceive, I had never realized how many adults were disgruntled at the infant and toddler shackles that barred them from entering movie theaters across America.

Movies, however, were not more important or vital to my life than having a baby. No date with Martin Scorsese, not even one jam-packed with blood, guns, and Jack Nicholson, could fill my void.

"You know," I said, stepping closer to Dr. GQ and placing my hand on his white-coated arm. "I've seen a lot of movies in my life, but I've never had a baby. I think it'll be a pretty fair trade. But I really do hope you get to see *The Departed* soon. That must be hard."

One squeeze of his forearm and I began my descent from Swedish Covenant Hospital. I called Constance on the way out to tell her the good news, to begin letting the world know that I wasn't the problem—that there was no problem.

On my drive home I stopped off at the video store to return *The Departed*, and later, we turned off the television and made love to hit the reset button and begin our three-month wait.

Chapter 10

• •

Testosterone, Kyle, and a Metaphoric Foot to the Groin

A flexible icepack, once used to maintain refrigerator temperature in a carton of soymilk on a drive from Peru to Chicago, was now nestled between my thighs on the sofa. Frozen peas were a decent substitute, but they defrosted and devolved into mush before my one-hour goal had been met and tended to make my private parts smell like an English pub. Ice in a baggie was a stupid idea, since it tended to leak onto the sheets through the cracks in the weak plastic, and the cut-to-size freezer pouches from the camping aisle at Target were too jagged for such a sensitive area. Those I only used while sitting at my desk at work, slyly removing a pouch from the unmarked brown bag in the freezer and whisking it off to the bathroom for proper placement.

Mom bought the extra lunchbox cooling packs as a means to keep food fresh on long drives. Pressed against my testicles, however, Mom's unintentional act of matronly love served me much better than anything else I could find to help lower the temperature of my bits.

Since we started over, giving our conception chances three more months before taking the next step, I had become even more diligent about my icing routine. Three more months to get it right wasn't the freedom Dr. GQ had intended. Instead, his suggestion felt like an ultimatum, a crazy ex-girlfriend stalking my every move, leaving lipstick-stained death threats on my windshield, signed "I'll love you forever." What our next step would be we didn't know, and the only proactive step I could take was upping my icing from one hour per day to two.

As the second hour of coldness came to a close, a frigid day in late February marching in with wind and snow to match my plummeting body temperature, my head was Caesar and my genitals Pompey, torn between the security of a peaceful Rome and the carnal urge to kick some ass and have sex. *The Golden Girls* reruns that were always on television were on again, but my eyes couldn't focus on the screen, and even if they had found solace in the moving images, I wouldn't have found joy in their innocent geriatric slapstick.

I wanted a steak, I wanted to throw Constance on the floor and kiss her chest and scratch my beard across her stomach, and I also wanted to bury my head beneath the purple throw pillows and cry about nothing. My hormone swings were worsening, and when the doorbell rang when no one was scheduled to drop by, I threw the remote control across the room and knocked over a pile of classics stacked vertically in the black lacquer bookcase.

"Who is it?" Constance shouted from the kitchen, in the midst of cleaning up the mess I had made while concocting a pot of lentil soup.

"How the hell should I know?" I fired back, not upset at her inquiry but with an unexpected interruption when my brain and body were cold and cranky strangers incapable of kindness. "Can you answer the door? I'm icing." Constance ran from the kitchen, sliding through the dining room across the hardwood floors until she reached the top of the stairs.

"Hello, Barhamand family!" Constance shouted. "Come on in! It's so good to see you guys. It's been forever."

Kyle, Holly, and Helena were known to stop by without notice because Helena was a doe-eyed handful, and Kyle's Trader Joe's schedule was constantly changing.

"Hey, Matty, what's up?" Kyle asked, running over to the sofa and hopping onto my lap. Wiry and small, Kyle was prone to throwing himself onto my broad back or into my arms, to play me like a jungle gym, and I loved playing his game. We were comic opposites, his black hair and my bald head, a foot of distance between the top of his head and mine, his first child conceived by chance and mine a constant struggle.

"Hey, Kyle. I'd get up but I'm icing my balls right now."

"Ewww," Holly said as Kyle jumped out of my arms and

took her coat, folding it in half and placing it over the back of a dining room chair. "I think I'll pass on the hug."

She was in the midst of becoming a trained doula and had offered to be there for the birth of our child if and when it happened. Holly knew more about pregnancy and childbirth than anybody I knew, a uterine encyclopedia, and had been trying to get Constance to monitor the viscosity of her vaginal mucus as a way of determining our fertile dates. Constance had yet to become a convert.

"How's that going?" Kyle asked. "Sounds like it must be fun for you down there."

"It's like sticking my junk in a snow bank," I said. "You should really give it a shot sometime. Maybe on your way home tonight."

Helena began to pull books off the shelf—Molly Ivins, Hemingway, and Camus—so in an effort to preserve our literature, I hopped up off the sofa, turned my back to our guests, and removed the ice pack from my pants. An hour and fifty-five minutes would have to suffice.

From the highest shelf in the bedroom closet, a shelf no one in the apartment could reach except me, I grabbed the blue plastic bin of stuffed animals and brought it into the living room. Helena and I ripped into the toys, tossing them into the air while Constance regaled our friends with stories of my urology visit. My brain was cramping and my crotch was thawing, and stringing words together into sentences for the bene-

READER/CUSTOMER CARE SURVEY

We care about your opinions! Please take a moment to fill out our online Reader Survey at **http://survey.hcibooks.com**.
As a **"THANK YOU"** you will receive a **VALUABLE INSTANT COUPON** towards future book purchases
as well as a **SPECIAL GIFT** available only online! Or, you may mail this card back to us.

(PLEASE PRINT IN ALL CAPS)

First Name _____ MI. _____ Last Name _____

Address _____ City _____

State _____ Zip _____ Email _____

1. Gender
□ Female   □ Male

2. Age
□ 8 or younger
□ 9-12   □ 13-16
□ 17-20   □ 21-30
□ 31+

3. Did you receive this book as a gift?
□ Yes   □ No

4. Annual Household Income
□ under $25,000
□ $25,000 - $34,999
□ $35,000 - $49,999
□ $50,000 - $74,999
□ over $75,000

5. What are the ages of the children living in your house?
□ 0 - 14   □ 15+

6. Marital Status
□ Single
□ Married
□ Divorced
□ Widowed

7. How did you find out about the book?
(please choose one)
□ Recommendation
□ Store Display
□ Online
□ Catalog/Mailing
□ Interview/Review

8. Where do you usually buy books?
(please choose one)
□ Bookstore
□ Online
□ Book Club/Mail Order
□ Price Club (Sam's Club, Costco's, etc.)
□ Retail Store (Target, Wal-Mart, etc.)

9. What subject do you enjoy reading about the most?
(please choose one)
□ Parenting/Family
□ Relationships
□ Recovery/Addictions
□ Health/Nutrition
□ Christianity
□ Spirituality/Inspiration
□ Business Self-help
□ Women's Issues
□ Sports

10. What attracts you most to a book?
(please choose one)
□ Title
□ Cover Design
□ Author
□ Content

TAPE IN MIDDLE; DO NOT STAPLE

ʰₐᵢₗₗₐₐᵢₗₗₐₐₗₐₗₐₗₐₗₗₐₗₗₗₗₐₗₐₗₐₗₐₗₐₐₗₗₐₗₐₗₐₗₐₗ

FOLD HERE

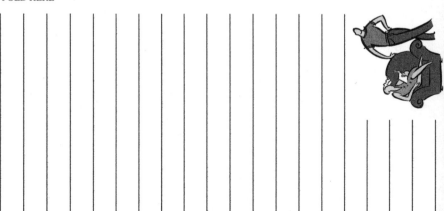

Comments

fit of my friends wasn't worth the effort to maintain niceties.

"Sorry if I'm being rude, you guys," I said. "My brain just isn't right from all of this."

As soon as I finished my sentence, a small brown teddy bear dressed in a bunny-rabbit onesie collided with my head. Every year my dad bought us each a stuffed animal for Christmas, an animal in which he saw a relative similarity— eyes, mouth, a tilt of the head—that captured our individualities. This Christmas, as a gift for our unconceived child, he picked out the bear that had just assaulted my head.

"Helena, no throwing," Holly said firmly, grabbing her daughter by the arm and swooping her up into her arms.

"So, this is bad timing, I know, with everything that's going on for you guys and the ice on your nuts, but it looks like we're going to have another one of these things in about seven months," Kyle said, pointing at Helena. His voice was usually a deep thunder, but he had dialed down his message with an apologetic softness.

"Wow, that's so great," I said, smiling in spite of the nauseating bomb of disappointment detonating in my throat. "I'm so happy for you guys."

Constance smiled and uttered a pained congratulations, but it was obvious to everyone in the room that our joy wasn't genuine, or at least not as voluptuous as the first time they had announced a pregnancy while in our living room. Balloons and wine and cake greeted the unmarried couple, terrified at the prospect of announcing their perceived indiscretion to strict families. Toasting Helena in her infancy was a reflex. My only reflex now, upon the announcement of their second child in three years, was to change the subject before one of us began to cry.

After they left, Constance and I didn't fill the emptiness with words, and I, for once, didn't try to joke my way back into normalcy. We crawled into bed and held each other between the Calvin Klein sheets that had begun to feel more and more like a stylishly worn liability that kept us from starting our family earlier. Back when it all could have been easier.

Chapter 11

· ·

The Third Time I Knew
I Wanted to Be a Father

Constance and I discussed having children for the first time during my junior year at the University of Iowa. We wouldn't be an official couple for another twelve months, but we spent night after night cuddled on my bed beneath the blue glow dripping from the Christmas lights strung around my bedroom. We listened to R.E.M., and I talked about my recent skin removal surgery to minimize the un-elastic skin that was left behind after my weight loss. Constance reminisced about spending her first semester in London and about the red phone booth from where she called me every day. I brushed my fingers through her hair. Constance ran her hands along the collar of my shirt, dipping her timid fingers onto my chest for moments so brief they were marked only by the shivers they sent down my ribs and into my groin.

We never once mentioned her confession of love via instant messenger from London—a confession that terrified me to the point of speechlessness and brought about a denied reciprocation of that love. It was a confession that defied my core belief that I was unlovable and that nobody who knew the real me—the remnants of the melted waxlike skin dripping from my body and hidden by my clothes—could gaze at my body and crave intercourse. A touch at the wrong time on a part of my body that made me feel abnormal gave me an excuse to pick a fight, to buy myself time before she saw what was hidden by my clothes. I knew that once she knew my body, she'd want nothing more to do with me. Nonetheless, by my junior year I knew that I wanted her to be the mother of my children, even if it meant a trip to the sperm bank to make it happen.

Junior year came and went, and we never once said, "I love you," but we repeatedly confessed to each other that we were the only people on Earth with whom we wanted to reproduce. Both of us wanted to have multitudes of Fumea-Miller babies together on an unspecified date in the distant future. We wanted to stick them with delightfully quirky monikers and instill in them a devotion to hipster indie rock and feminist anarchy. Sex was never part of that discussion.

One year later, by the time we had stopped the bickering that had emerged from unfulfilled sexual tension and officially began to date, it was all afternoon make-out excursions to movie theaters and local botanical gardens, and every thought of children was an inevitability. But it wasn't something we desired until we had secured graduate degrees and high-paying jobs. I overcame my body issues, and for the first time in my life I was able to be both intimate and in love with the same person.

"I'm afraid, sometimes, about being a father," I said the night after our cold war ended, the day we began to date, and the makeshift wall separating the east and west sides of our room came billowing down. At the beginning of my senior year we moved into a farm-style house with our friend Lisa Weimar and my best friend Sarah Schmitt, and Constance and I shared a giant bedroom. One day, when the aforementioned sexual tension dissolved into outright tension, I strung a wire down the center of the room and pinned a sheet to it. Once I allowed her to judge my body for herself, once I stopped punishing her for my shame, the love that I had pressurized since my junior year finally blew-up in my face. And I had never felt more whole.

"You'll be a great dad someday," she said. "Why are you afraid?"

"If I have a kid that ends up being fat, I'll never forgive myself. I don't want to pass that on to another child, another person that has to go through what I've gone through in my life. I can't pass on my issues to someone else."

In many facets of health I viewed myself as an enormous success: a thin, two-hundred-ten-pound, toned athlete. On several levels, though, I continued to fail myself daily. Neither an apple nor apple pie could cross my lips without excessive deliberation, guilt, and careful planning that was also accompanied by loathing. Every time I saw someone running or walking, even if I had already run eight miles that day, I wanted to pull the car to the side of the road and take off at a sprint.

"That doesn't have to happen," Constance said, lowering her head onto my chest. I flexed my pectoral muscles to create the illusion I was in even better shape than I was. "We won't let that happen. It's totally in our control."

"I know that," I said. "I suppose I don't believe in myself yet. At least not to the point where I feel like an adequate role model. If my childhood was Antarctica, I want my kid grow up in Tahiti. I want his or her life to be the total opposite of mine."

It all came to a head that morning during my run through the residential neighborhoods of Iowa City en route to the river. Hoards of families were beginning their days. Parents shuffling kids down the street with their Spiderman backpacks and Barbie tennis shoes bouncing in time with the pace of my feet. Minivans filling up with children lamenting their hate of entry-level education, and nearly every parent clutching a coffee mug as if it were the nectar of life that kept them from dragging their pokey children by the arm and into the vehicle.

Pangs of jealousy pricked me in anticipation of my own future routine, for the day when I would take a hybrid version of Constance and me, decked out in an R.E.M. T-shirt, to elementary school. But around mile six, while passing the eighth obese woman I had seen accompanied by her obese children, my windpipe closed up and my already-heaving chest seized. The sweat stinging my eyes was replaced by the sting of tears.

I don't want a fat kid, I thought. *I'm going to mess this all up for them, just like I did for myself.*

I stopped running to hold court with a panic attack outside of Phillips Hall, which by that time of day was experiencing an influx of red-eyed students stuck with a class that had the audacity to commence before ten. Head between my legs, I stretched my palms downward and placed them flat on the ground. I was taking deep breaths and struggling to recover from the grief of seeing heredity played out in front of my eyes, like the pages of a how-not-to manual come to life.

And then as I took off running, I failed to notice the obstruction now in front of me, and I fell face first into a bush as a group of frat boys walked by.

"Dude, did you see that? That was awesome. That dude just biffed into the bush!"

I rolled onto my butt in the center of the unforgiving shrubbery and swatted away the blood and leaves that clung to my legs. I pulled myself up with the aid of the black metal railing lining the ramp next to the walkway as the boys disappeared into Phillips Hall for what I hoped was an eternity and future of fatness.

Easter Sunday 1995 flashed through my head as I continued

to grip the railing, a flipbook of Chelsey's lighted sneakers, the sparkling premonitions of my death trailing behind her, and the realization I wanted to live long enough to be a father. Animated in my mind, slow-motion stills of that day sprang back to life during a moment when I barely had the courage to pull myself up from a fall that dropped me in the presence of boys who made me feel inferior. I was weak, but what was worse was that I knew how weak I was, and despite that, I still had one inescapable thought: *at least my kid won't be a frat boy*.

Genes that potentially could be passed from me to my child continued to occupy every parental notion I had for the foreseeable thereafter, but it didn't make me want to be a father any less. In fact, it seemed like the only opportunity I might have to redo the segment of my life I had squandered. I couldn't reclaim time, but through my child I could get a picture of what my body and my childhood could have been minus the weight. And despite my obesity concerns I couldn't wait for that snapshot to develop.

Chapter 12

- -

Endocrines, Dr. Leya,
and the Intrepid "I" Word

"Reproductive" had long been a dutiful soldier in my army of words. Apparently, "endocrinologist" had remained a conscientious objector, skipping the daily battles of word wit with my fellow Content That Works editors to sip martinis along the shores of my left brain. Its moment of leisure, and with it my reproductive innocence, was about to come to an abrupt end. Three months after my clean bill of sperm health (three months after hitting the reset button that reset nothing), we decided it was Constance's turn to be evaluated. I turned to my blog friends to ask the more experienced "infertiles" what our next step should be. We knew a fertility specialist of some breed was needed, but neither of us was sure what term to search under on our insurance's website to find the appropriate practitioner for our needs. Before I could finish my post in order to collect some free advice, an e-mail from Constance dropped into my inbox. "We need a reproductive

endocrinologist," Constance e-mailed me from her work station while I remained at home, blogging from the sofa. "I did some searching on other people's blogs and it seems like that's who we need to see. Do you have time to find the one closest to us? I don't care who it is, I just don't want to travel a long way to every appointment. From what I've heard, we'll be going there a lot. If you find one, I'll set up the appointment."

Dr. Joan Leya was one of two doctors in all of Chicago who was covered by our plan, and her office in south Evanston was close enough to our apartment and a Starbucks to make repeat trips manageable. Evanston was where Constance and I wanted to move once our children were of school-age. It had better schools and a wider-aisle Whole Foods. It seemed logical that perhaps Evanston was the preeminent destination to get that future kick-started, so I e-mailed Dr. Leya's contact information to Constance and went back to writing a new entry in my blog.

Ten minutes later another e-mail from Constance appeared with instructions for our first visit, which was scheduled to occur in two days' time.

"She says we should just come any time between six and eight in the morning!" Constance wrote. "Have you ever heard of a doctor's office opening so early? That will make getting to work so much easier!"

I closed the lid of my laptop without saving my current work, slamming the MacBook against the coffee table, and closing my eyes to seal the gap between Constance's message and my impending freak-out. From the bedroom to the outside world, it was another landmark on our trip from normal sex to assisted reproduction, and one that was uncomfortably close to the final destination. I wanted to be happy about moving forward, and I wanted to be angry about the same thing, so instead I turned up the volume on the television and allowed news of the previous day's sports scores to lull me to sleep.

The next night, before band practice, Constance and I heated up some butternut squash soup and spread a thick layer of goat cheese on two pieces of bread and sat at the dining-room table.

"So, how are you feeling about tomorrow?" I asked, dipping my finger into the excess goat cheese and clumping it on the end of my finger.

"I'm nervous, I guess," she said. "I'm never excited to get weighed or to have a stranger poking around inside of me."

I smeared the goat cheese across my upper lip like a moustache and flashed Constance the broadest smile possible.

"Do you remember that time at Chili's," she laughed, "when you put sour cream and guacamole all over your face right before the waitress came to take our plates?"

During college I had taken to slathering food on my face or putting uneaten bread bowls on my bald head. Composure maintained, I would ask the confused server for more soda or to direct me to the bathroom, at which point I would strut through the restaurant with crappy chain cuisine on my brow.

"You know, all of these people on my blog told us to go see an RE," I said, shaving my faux-cheese moustache off with my tongue. "And so, without question I went to our insurance website, found our two options, and before I knew it, you had made an appointment less than two days from now. I don't even know what a reproductive endocrinologist is, and if you do, please don't tell me. I want to be surprised."

"Why didn't you just look it up on the Web?"

"Because . . . I have no good reason, that's why. I'm fully prepared to walk into that office tomorrow and ask our doctor if she can point me in the general direction of where my endocrine is located."

"Please, don't do that," Constance said, laughing at what I'm sure she thought was another episode of my facetious routine, but in reality was a routine I was fully prepared to entertain if the tension got too thick and bitter for me to swallow.

"I'm taking my camera, too, just like I did on our urologist visit. Just in case we get some good shots for the blog."

"I'm glad you're coming with me," Constance said, reaching across the table, tickling her fingers across the top of my hands. "Dr. Leya said only about ten percent of husbands come to these appointments with their wives or partners."

"That's bullshit," I said, as I leaned forward and kissed each one of Constance's fingers. "This isn't just for you or about you, this is for us. I'm just as much a part of this as you, baby."

⌐～～⌐

Dr. Leya's practice was in an unassuming office on the third floor of Resurrection Hospital, a space completely void of paint and style. A small beaded portrait of what looked to be a Native American woman was the only frivolous addition to the congregation of conventional waiting-room chairs and stacks of magazines.

"Hello! Just sign the sheet and have a seat. I'll be with you in a few minutes," a voice shouted from behind a plain vanilla-covered wall dissected by an unmarked door and a tiny drive-through window.

I plopped down in a chair and popped open an outdated issue of *Vogue* that promised to guide me toward can't-miss hotness for 2006, a year too late to be a guiding principle for the year to come. Posited on the final page of the publication was one of those ironic question-and-answer sessions with celebrities; the incredulous interviewer asks a series of non-sequiturs to delve into the mind of a creative "genius."

What always happens, however, is the celebrity in question ends up sounding pompous, arrogant, and self-aggrandizing by responding to a question such as "If you were to be rein-carnated, what would you want to be in the next life?" with an answer as infuriating as "A lime tree." Which is what French actress Catherine Deneuve said, and in my anxious state, it was more than enough stupid to set me off on a tirade.

"Yeah, I hope you have an enlightening journey segueing from a renowned actress lazing away your afternoons on the French Riviera, sipping champagne in your Yves St. Laurent dress into an immobile, bark-covered, bitter fruit tree," I said.

"What are you talking about?" Constance asked, lowering her home-decorating magazine and raising her voice, a sword to my ranting throat. First impressions were vital to my wife, and she didn't want Dr. Leya to get the right impression about my quirky peculiarities.

"Catherine Deneuve says she wants to be reincarnated as a lime tree. A lime tree! What crap. You know what? I hope she gets her wish. I hope she has a nice time with that, and I hope her lime tree is in some rural area where lots of animals and people pee all over her every day."

My nerves were manifesting in anger, and it didn't help that earlier in the interview this flawless woman confessed that her least favorite body part was her left ear. Normal people have bigger fish to fry than something as innocent as an ear. Catherine Deneuve provided me a shore on which my emotional hurricane could make destructive contact before we met our reproductive endocrinologist for the first time.

"Hi, I'm Dr. Leya," said a petite middle-aged woman who poked her head through the tiny window in the wall—a taller infertility equivalent to the guard at the entrance of Emerald City.

Her blond hair was pulled back, like a tennis player's, into a tight ponytail that wouldn't move whether hitting a forehand down the line or scurrying around a delivery room. Simply dressed in a white smock, no makeup or flashy accessories, she was a natural woman who looked like a cross between Mother Earth and a suffragette.

"Come on back and we'll get started," she said.

Constance and I stood up, placed our magazines back on the pile, and followed the blue Berber carpet, finally heading off to see the Wizard of Vag.

We sat down in front of her desk in chairs that matched those in the waiting room. Her office was cluttered, but it was obvious that the piles and stacks of books were an organized system from which she could retrieve information at will.

"So, why are you guys here?"

At this point, our story was a comedy routine, a back-and-forth exchange of upbeat lines that divulged our predicament with the verve usually reserved for stand-up. Our lines were memorized and our timing perfect. It was a routine so well rehearsed that I no longer had to worry myself with the content of the message. Performing allowed us to skip the picking at an open wound that a heartfelt confession required.

"Did you bring copies of your semen analysis?" she asked, looking up from the second page of notes she had scribbled during our monologues.

"Yes," I said. "The doctor did two, and here are both. One

had a count of ten million and the other was sixty million. The only thing that wasn't right was my pH, and I don't know if that is something we should look into further or not."

"I tend not to worry about a slightly elevated pH or one low count," she said, handing my sperm printouts back to me. "Counts vary, and getting one in the really high range is great. We can officially put your sperm to bed."

The muscles in my face were stronger than the will of my brain, and I couldn't bury the adolescent smile blooming on my face. Bred partially of relief but mostly of childishness, my infantile sensibilities still found her blunt comments and choice of words an oversized popsicle in the mouth of a pretty girl.

"Constance, do you have regular periods?"

"Yes," she said, grabbing my hand. I squeezed her tiny palm, and she wiggled free from my grip. Dr. Leya's questions were fingers poking my chest, and her routine inquiry into my wife's most private functions elevated my blood pressure.

"How long do you bleed?"

"My cycle is usually twenty-eight days, Constance said. "My period usually lasts about five days."

"Have you had any go longer than that since you've been trying."

"A couple," she said, her voice cracking and softening, showing the weakness of the one ten-day near miss that was the closest we made it to pregnancy. "I had one period that was ten days late, but I've never had a positive pregnancy test."

After walking Constance through a litany of medical-history questions—no family history of breast or ovarian cancer, a recent family history of colon cancer and thyroid troubles—Dr. Leya said there was nothing on the surface that looked to be of note.

"And the good news is you're young," she said. "I get so many people in here who are pushing forty, and when you're old, you're old. You guys at least have good sperm and youth on your side."

Straight talk was refreshing, and Dr. Leya didn't sugarcoat or soften her words or her tone. She talked to us like a directive parent, and it was exactly the aggressive guidance we craved in the sea of positive blindness we received from our loved ones. Dr. Leya admitted, however, that a couple in such good health and at our tender age should be pregnant by now.

"We'll get your infertility solved," she said. "During your next menstrual cycle, provided you don't get pregnant this cycle, you'll come in for a series of five tests at different points, including a pelvic x-ray on day eight to kick off the festivities. Today you'll head down to the lab for blood tests. I want to test your follicle-stimulating hormone, your prolactin and estrogen and testosterone levels, as well as your blood type. If you're a negative and Matt is a positive that could be our answer."

Her list continued, but I still was caught in the net of her first statement. Dr. Leya's words weren't explicit; she didn't come right out and say we were infertile, but by promising to solve our infertility, she was labeling us as such for the first time. Our lack of success no longer felt like a frustrating inconvenience. It officially was a problem with a medical name prescribed by a medical professional.

Constance shed no tears in the office, and I had no inappropriate outbursts, but after we left her office to head to the lab for blood tests, Constance burrowed into my arms and we held each other as the elevator doors opened and closed repeatedly, intermittently bathing us in an artificial glow before slamming with a jarring, metronomic click. Both of us were teary and head cramped, like a rainy day when the elevated barometric pressure fills your sinuses and you feel like you've been sucking on a helium tap.

"It's really real now," Constance said. "It feels weird to have a doctor tell you it was the right thing to come to her. Oh, and to hear her say we are infertile! That means we definitely have a problem. It's very real now."

Not once during our visit did I think to reach for my camera, nor did I remember to ask for directions to my endocrine. It was very real, and it was very intimate. Having someone ask my wife, "How long do you bleed?" curdled my anger. I couldn't help but vacillate between feeling violated and overjoyed, between longing to hug this woman and throw her out the third-floor window.

After the needles drew their information from Constance's

veins, we left the hospital and went home, skipping work for the rest of the day to watch reruns of *Arrested Development* and allow ourselves to process our newfound status as infertiles.

Infertile. We were infertile. Constance was due to ovulate the following week, and this cycle would be our last chance to get pregnant the normal way—without assistance and without medication. It was our last chance to escape the label of "infertile" and get the job done ourselves.

⁓

Constance's ovaries obviously had a sense of humor, a Sarah Silverman–style inappropriateness, or else they wouldn't have placed us in separate twin beds fewer than fifty feet from my in-laws' bedroom on egg-delivery weekend for what would be our final all-natural sex week.

In the flurry and fury of modern air travel, I had forgotten that we were due for an egg drop, which is something I'd been closely monitoring over the past year. After our visit with Dr. Leya, we both shifted our focus to thoughts of conception in the future, as if a few pelvic exams and blood analyses would blow the whistle on our stalemate. We didn't lend credence to the possibility that the month at hand would be *the* month. We had stopped believing in our ability to create a child the old-fashioned, down-home way.

But even proper Southern decency and thin walls could not

keep us from our goal. With my feet hanging off the short twin bed, we made love for the last normal time—just very, very quietly so as not to disturb the silent house or the nervous collie dog pacing the hallways.

Down in North Carolina life moved at a slower pace. Constance's parents, Richard and Susan, wanted to go to the racetrack for breakfast, my least favorite place to eat in all of Pinehurst, and the slow service following my morning run meant my bowl of lumpy oatmeal didn't arrive until my hunger-induced headache had already begun to throb. At every square table—each one covered by a dingy plastic tablecloth—were men dressed in polo shirts sans popped-collars (we city folk flip for fun) and women with open-toed shoes and toenails painted a pink so pastel that I was overcome by an urge to gather their toes like Easter eggs.

Later that day, Richard and Susan opened their arms and six bottles of wine to separate our minds from infertility via familial inebriation. We sat outside on the enclosed porch overlooking soaring pine trees and the flooded ravine flowing through their backyard and told them for the first time, on Mother's Day, the details of our baby-making woes. I handed Susan a stack of printed pages, my entire blog in physical form to give my mother-in-law an inside look into what Constance and I had been going through.

"On Friday I told my boss about our infertility because I'm going to be taking so much time off for doctor appointments," Constance said, sipping her third glass of the home-made red wine that Richard and his executive buddies cooked up in a suburban Chicago basement. "And do you know what she said? '*Congratulations*.' She paused for a second and then said, 'I mean, on thinking about expanding your family, not about the other stuff.' She's a truly nice woman, and in an effort to uphold the dignity of her position while infusing it with a sisterly warmth, she said 'congratulations' when I told her I'm infertile. This whole process has been so bizarre and frustrating, Mom."

"Well, if it's any consolation, I'm still menstruating, and I'm fifty-four," Susan said as a thunderclap boomed behind her intimate confession, the humid afternoon turning even more airless after hearing word of my mother-in-law's continuing menstruation.

"Gee, thanks," Constance said, equally repulsed by the ideas of aged parenthood and eternal menstruation. I was repulsed simply by the idea of my mother-in-law's menstrual cycle.

As Susan read the printed pages of my blog in reverse from the newest entry to the oldest because her carpal-tunnel-stricken hand couldn't handle the strain of computer use, she looked up with tears in her eyes and said, "Constance, I'm so sorry you've had to deal with this."

"Thank you, Mom. It's not easy."

"You guys will find your way," Richard said, swirling his goblet counter-clockwise to measure the legs of his wine.

"And if not, you have other options," Susan said. "Take the drugs and do what you need to do. That's what they're there for."

"Thank you, Susan," I said, walking over to hold her in my arms and thank her for her sincerity and for not excusing our problems away. "Having such great support from the both of you will make this a lot easier on us."

"You know what's great about this writing," Susan said, the soft skin of her pale face still pressed against my cheek, "is that on the surface it's about your infertility, but, Constance, these are all love letters to you."

Constance placed her hand down the back of my pants and stroked my lower back.

"I love you," I whispered.

"I love you," she said.

"And don't let us stop you from trying this weekend. I just read that you're ovulating. You can push those beds together if you need to."

"I'll help you," Richard said, as we all burst into unexpected laughter in unison with the thunder, which began to crack as a light rain started to seep through the mesh walls of the porch.

Chapter 13

· ·

Peanut, Doulas, and Tears in a Des Moines Hospital

Moments ticked by excruciatingly slowly as always that Friday morning, the emerging May tulips and rising temperatures an Eden of temptation for the white-collar set. Unlike most workweek finales, however, my unhealthy stalking of the clock was paparazzi caliber, knowing that the intoxicating chug of the secondhand could, at any minute, send my sister Angie into labor and ignite the birthing process for the precious girl my family had taken to calling Peanut.

Visions of Peanut's unknowable mug occupied my fantasies, and between resizing high-resolution photos for Web use and updating the health-and-wellness site under my command, I pictured a newborn baby with my sister's head and interchanged her body parts, first applying the Miller family tree-trunk thighs and then the Johnson family stick legs. On her scalp I placed a mop of reddish-blond hair like her father's and then exchanged it in favor of an uncontrollable nest of dark brown like her mother's. "Neon Bible" thumped in my headphones, and I wondered if Peanut would emerge from the womb a Nickleback fan like her mother or perhaps bestowed with the more refined tastes of an Arcade Fire devotee like her uncle.

I wondered these things on behalf of Peanut, but I was really imagining my own child sporting a Rilo Kiley onesie and a faux-hawk, with Constance's perfect blue eyes and my button nose, with my musical sensibilities and Constance's social activism. This was the moment I wanted to have for myself, a moment of possibility that through the violent, nauseating miracle of childbirth, my son or daughter would take root in the real world and be everything I had hoped for and more.

I had been present for the birth of all of my nieces and nephews, and I was going to be there for Peanut, too, even though her arrival would take place in a hospital over six hours away. Angie, due to her high-risk pregnancy and because her first child was born via Cesarean, had scheduled her C-section the week before Chelsey's fifteenth birthday. Constance and I scheduled vacation days to stay with Chelsey and her stepbrother, Sabastian, to take care of them while Angie and Junior stayed with their newborn. We planned to drive to Iowa City the night before in order to be at the hospital in Des Moines by seven AM.

Like all good plans, however, they momentarily jumped the shark when my sister peed her pants—twice.

"Well, your sister thinks her water broke at work this morning," Mom said, breathing heavily into the telephone as if she were calling me from the cockpit of her fighter jet. "She had to change her underwear twice, and then Junior came to work and picked her up and took her to the hospital."

"Should I be getting on the road right now?" I asked, closing my laptop lid halfway in anticipation her answer would be "yes." "I don't want to miss this, Mom!"

"Honey, I don't know. Angie said she'd call as soon as she knows anything, and then I'll let you know."

Constance and I were held captive, not clear whether to run home and pack the car or continue on with work as usual. After two hours of waiting and two Venti coffees, and after mentally whipping myself for the physical distance I had placed between me and my niece-in-waiting that would keep me from greeting her at the moment she waltzed from the womb, Mom called again.

"False alarm," she said, her voice now calm and absent of worried breaths. "It looks like she either has a small leak in the fluid sac, or a urinary tract infection that, well, caused her to be a little backed up."

"You mean she peed her pants?" I asked, laughing both in relief and at the expense of my incontinent sister, my heart racing from the excessive caffeine and adrenaline of a quasi-birth.

"Well, maybe. They don't know what caused it for sure, but essentially, yes. Your sister peed her pants. But it's not a baby, so the scheduled C-section is still on for Wednesday."

"So, did you or did you not pee your pants today?" I asked. After work we made a quick bite to eat as the excitement built, for the first time in my life, to make a phone call and utter the aforementioned phrase.

"Shut up!" Angie said, snorting as her laugh went from a steady chuckle to a silent heave.

"It's cool. I wee myself a little from time to time. We once saw a segment on TV when Liv Tyler admitted that one time she peed her pants a little bit. Maybe you're just Steven Tyler's long-lost daughter."

"No, it wasn't really pee," she said, struggling to catch her breath. "Well, not mine anyway. Either Peanut's mucus plug came loose, or there's a small leak at the very top of my water sac. When Junior was driving me to the hospital, I was so worried I wouldn't have time to wash our sheets so you and Constance would have a clean bed to sleep in while you're watching the kids."

"I'm just so thankful we'll get to be there," I said, no jealousy or thoughts of what I was missing clouding my relief. "It would have killed me to miss this big moment for you. I'm just so happy."

"Me, too," Angie said. "I'm just not quite ready."

"I think you're ready," I said. "You're peeing your pants with excitement, what more could you want?"

Scene: A modest-size, well-decorated Chicago bathroom on the afternoon of Saturday, May 19. The sun is shining through the vented window inside the shower, casting a nauseating glow upon Matthew, who looks like he was recently run over by several trucks after a night sipping copious amounts of red wine. Constance, preparing to shower, is pressing her nose into the vanity mirror, inspecting her manicured eyebrows for strays.

Matthew: Woah!

Constance: What?

Matthew: Well, if I'm being completely honest, your boobs look bigger.

Constance: Really? Are you sure?

Matthew: Yes, they are definitely popping out the top of your bra a bit.

Constance: Ouch! They feel swollen and really tender, like when I get swollen glands in my neck.

Matthew: What do you think it means?

Constance: Nope, I'm not going there. I'm not even entertaining that thought. I refuse to get my hopes up.

Matthew: MayoClinic.com says it's the first sign of pregnancy.

Constance: You know, you'd think my first thought would be positive, like 'yeah, maybe I'm pregnant,' but if we got pregnant this month, at my parents' house, then we'd be 'proving' my mom right, and I'd never hear the end of it.

Matthew: What do you mean?

Constance: She said we just needed to get away for the weekend and relax in North Carolina and we'd get pregnant. I think she thinks that I'm too stressed to get pregnant, but I'm not stressed. God, if this were to happen I'd never hear the end of it.

Matthew: God, you're right. She'd totally take the credit for it, and she'd start talking about how we need to live quieter, less complicated lives like Christopher Robin and Winnie-the-Pooh. Then we'd have to start having tea parties with cucumber sandwiches every single day before retiring to the study to read Dickens and watching *Masterpiece Theatre*.

Constance: Why does it bug me to prove my mom right? That's sick! I'm a terrible daughter.

Matthew: Because in your mind it will invalidate our problem in her mind. As if the problem wasn't medical, but due to the fact we just needed to relax. But the truth is, if tenderness and swelling is baby related, it probably happened before our trip to North Carolina anyway. Besides, it's probably nothing, but I do have to say again, they are noticeably bigger.

Constance: Oh, no! They don't have that nice up-slope anymore. What is going on? This has *never* happened to me before.

Matthew: I'm sure it's nothing, but having said that, if you wanted to take a pregnancy test, I wouldn't say no.

Constance: No, not until Thursday.

Matthew: I hate feeling hopeful. Boobs used to be way more fun before they became pregnancy predictors.

Constance: Ugh! Now my hopes are up. I guess it was inevitable. But it's probably nothing. Ouch, they're really sore. I'm gonna look like Pam Anderson if this keeps up.

End scene.

One line, one bright pink column, and nothing more. We couldn't wait until Thursday. We needed to know whether or not we were pregnant before going into the birthing wing, where emotions and estrogen would be raging at a fevered pitch. Breasts, like all wonderful-yet-imperfect things, lie from time to time, and apparently one of the PMS symptoms that Constance never before had suffered decided to rear its ugly head to bring us false hope in a time when we were looking for the real thing.

"I'm sure seeing the new baby and wondering if we were next would have made the fallout all the more painful," Constance said, wiping her eyes again as she sat on the toilet, waiting five minutes for failure. "Now at least we can deal with our disappointment before we share in Angie's joy."

"It's still going to be hard," I said, kneeling down in front of the toilet. My face level to Constance's, I could see the redness coloring the whites of her eyes and the wet impression of tears that had dried on her pale cheeks like translucent varicose veins. "We'll get through it together. Even if your boobs are liars."

"Stupid boobs," she said, laughing and sniffling the remnants of her frustration back inside her body, saving it for the next time the test refused to produce dual lines.

～⌘～

Lurking inches away from the glass as a nurse probed, poked, flipped, and inked my newborn niece like a plainclothes cop booking our little Aliyah for excessive cuteness, the core of my family—Mom, Dad, April, Chelsey, Sabastian, Constance, and I—united in ogling its newest member.

Constance stood in front of me and I wrapped my arms around her, sensing that the abundance of love and adoration, the banter between everyone except us—which family member was responsible for providing Aliyah those deep blue eyes, her soft round nose, and a nonexistent butt—was segueing from joy to unflattering despair.

"If I were Angie, I'd be going crazy without my baby right now," I said, looping my finger through a perfect brown curl bouncing like a pliable spring against Constance's blushed cheek.

"Do you think she even got to hold her?" Constance asked, squeezing my wrists in a heartbeat cadence, quickening as thoughts of natal injustice bent her shape from jealous to furious. Too many mothers aren't given the power or respect they deserve in the delivery rooms, and our friend Holly, now a fully-licensed doula, had put the bug in Constance's ear about what was best for mother and child. Angie's best interests, she feared, were not being considered, and the hospital's denial of immediate bonding time, their assembly-line treatment of mother and child, wasn't sitting well.

"I doubt it," I said. "I think they brought Aliyah straight here for some reason. It would be so hard to go through that and then spend the first hour of your baby's life in separate rooms."

"Well, that's crap," she said. "We're going to have a doula when we get pregnant because I don't want to be pushed around by the hospital and have decisions made based on what is easiest for the doctor. Unless there's something wrong with the baby there is no need to rush it out here for all of this."

"Yeah, this just won't work for me. I'll have a nice little chat with our doctor when the time comes. Don't you worry."

Constance looked up at me, her eyes glistening with tears, and I embraced her tighter. Under any normal circumstance a liberal rant of this magnitude wouldn't have taken place in the presence of my parents, but with a new grandchild and a new digital camera, they were too occupied with the beauties of science and technology to hear our critique.

A stack of *People* magazines were piled at our feet, gifts from our friend Lisa who routinely lifted back issues from her mother's dermatology office and dropped them on us in ten-pound, three-month supplies. On the cover at the top of the stack was a picture of a heavily made-up Marcia Cross, airbrushed and glowing like a rash, clutching her new twin babies. Two more new babies flowed into the postbirthing room, a boy and a girl, and between the three infants in my presence and the two in Marcia Cross's bony arms, my breakfast of orange juice, coffee, and a Clif bar began a fist-fight in my stomach. After forty-five minutes in front of the glass, watching Aliyah scream and my family swoon, we needed a break from Marcia Cross and all of the flagrant baby flaunting occurring in the three-foot radius surrounding our embrace.

"We're going to go get something to drink," I announced, grabbing Constance by the hand and walking her toward the electronic doorway.

"Okay, Matthew," Mom said, her eyes locked on Aliyah and her head tilting only far enough for me to make out the corner of her mouth. "I'll have my cell on in case you come back and we're not here anymore."

I hit the exit button and the automatic doors purred, pulling open to reveal a new set of anxious relatives taking up residence where we had gathered at seven that morning.

"Good luck and congratulations," I said to a man who was about to be a new grandfather or an incredibly old father.

"Thanks," he said, bursting out of his worry and speaking

in the hoarse voice of someone who hadn't spoken to another living person in a few hours. "We should know something any minute."

Constance and I walked toward the floating glass staircase. Des Moines's new birthing unit was ultramodern, the hallways lined with avant-garde art, and it was precisely the kind of place I would have chosen to have our baby had it not been for the location. I stopped on the second step of the down staircase to even the height difference between Constance and me and pulled her into my arms.

"This is so hard," she said, her lips colliding with my earlobe, the harshness of her vowels pushing a steady air current against my cheek. "I'm so happy for Angie, but I'm tired of waiting. Where's our baby?"

"We'll get there, sweetie," I said. "At least we have a plan in action. You're going for your first test in a week, and I feel like we're closer to a solution than we've ever been."

"If there is a solution."

"Well, let's take a look at all the good things we already know. We know my sperm is okay and that you are more than capable of ovulating. That's more than some people can say, and until somebody tells me differently, I have to believe our functioning parts will someday yield an offspring."

"I know that, but this is all just a little harder than I imagined," she said.

"Yeah, for me, too."

After an extended embrace, we walked down the remaining stairs and out the front doors of the hospital. One full loop around the premises on foot, and we didn't see a single baby for twenty consecutive minutes: adequate tot-free time to revitalize the infertile spirit in the face of a glorious day of celebration, to spend a day honoring the expansion of my immediate family without the fear of crying for our immediate baby needs.

Chapter 14

. . . .

Iodine E-mail from
Daughter to Mother

Hi Mom!

Thanks for calling today—it was really sweet of you. I would have totally called you yesterday, but it was a really horrible, long day—I had to go to work after the test (which I shouldn't have done) b/c I was out so much of last week to go to Iowa, and I had a night meeting that would have been a huge pain to reschedule. I had an x-ray of my uterus done yesterday morning, which involves them injecting iodine and shoving all sorts of fun things around inside me. The test dyes your uterus and fallopian tubes to see if there is any blockage. My Dr. didn't see any at the time, but a more in-depth analysis is done for growths, etc., after the fact.

If you read about the test it says there may be some "mild cramping." All I have to say is mild cramping my ass! First of all, it's not cramping, it's pain.

Second of all, it's not mild. A work friend of mine who went through this wrote me today and said, "My nurse practitioner had that test done, and she told them she was going to pass out from the pain. They said 'You can't pass out, you're lying down,' and she said' Oh, yes, I can.' I believe we are all horribly mislead about the pain involved in that procedure. Honestly, giving birth (with an epidural of course) was way less painful." I quote her because that about sums it up. At least the pain wasn't for too long—probably three to five minutes, but I might not be a good judge of the time. Bleh!

Then, of course, three hours later I had a reaction to the iodine and developed a hot itchy rash that looked and felt exactly like a sunburn all over my torso, chest, neck, and back. I took a lot of Benadryl and it went away, but now the doctor says I will always have to tell doctors about my reaction b/c they use it in surgeries so much AND I may now be allergic to shellfish. Apparently, they are one and the same allergy and the high dose of iodine may have unleashed an allergy to iodine in shellfish. Geez! My next test is on Monday to check the health of my mucus, which should be like exams I'm used to. What a crazy process.

Iowa was good, but the first day was hard because it's very awkward to feel happy and sad at the same time. We got through it pretty well, and I think Angie understood because she battled infertility for YEARS before this baby was born. Actually the worst part of the trip was that a weather service alarm woke us up one morning to a flash flood. We had to pump the basement for more than six hours! In good news, baby Aliyah (or Ali, as Matt and I call her) is gorgeous and doing well. Check out Matt's blog for pics.

Love you and glad you are coming to visit in June!

C

Chapter 15

. . . .

Postcoital, Misconceptions, and a Room for Baby

Some tests, like those administered by the DMV, cause trepidation mostly because they are a time-suck, and the test givers tend to be disgruntled, unfriendly folk ready to rail you for even the slightest misstep, or for not being able to recall with certainty how far away from a two-way stop one should initiate the turning signal if a cement truck is parked diagonally on the opposing one-way street.

Others, such as aptitude tests, stir one part anxiety with two parts doubt and one part unprepared to concoct a toxic elixir that determines how smart or dumb one is based on calculating the circumference of something obtuse.

None of those tests that have assessed us from childhood to adulthood have equaled the pressure of the Monday morning in June when we set the alarm for five in the morning, put the dog in her crate, made love as the sun rose over Lake Michigan, and drove to Evanston for a postcoital exam.

"Now, I just want to make sure, because I've heard differing claims, but is a postcoital exam really necessary?" Constance asked, her hair damp and darker than usual, her face a pinpricked, deflating balloon. Once again seated in Dr. Leya's office, three days before we were to have our intimacy judged by a panel of experts, we held hands and held out hope that we could have sex on Monday morning and fall back to sleep per our normal postcoital routine. Neither of us was anxious to orgasm and run, and neither of us was ready to receive news that we had been doing it wrong all of these years. Sex was a delicious instinct, but it was about to become a gymnastics competition, and everything from our floor routine to the dismount would be scrutinized.

I didn't want to find out I was a bad lover from our doctor.

"You know, some say yes and some say no," Dr. Leya said. "I do it as a matter of course just to cross one more issue off the list. Sometimes the vagina can be a hostile place for semen, and this way I can get a good swab test to make sure there is a sufficient number of sperm alive within an hour after you have sex."

"Do you have to carry her upside down to the hospital?" my friend Tim joked later that day at work. Tim was a typical dude, your run-of-the-mill stoner with curly hair and threadbare clothes, only he had never smoked marijuana in his life. After he was hired we quickly became inappropriate friends, trading instant-messaged barbs in a relentless seesaw battle to be more inappropriate, disgusting, and shocking than the other.

"No, but I should totally do it anyway and see what the doctor says," I said, holding my Venti coffee in one hand and pretending to throw Constance over my shoulder with the other. "'We're here for our postcoital exam. Just did her in the car and brought her right in. What? Oh, really? I guess we misunderstood the directions. Sorry!'"

"Dude, you should just whip it out and start going at it right there in her office, on the exam table," he said, taking a sip from the always present Diet Mountain Dew next to his computer monitor. "It's no stranger than what you have to do in reality, and it would serve her right for trying to get a piece of your action."

Later that night at band practice we gave Jenni and Kamila their weekly update on our infertility, which had become as big a part of our practices as making music. Plugging cords into practice amps and tuning guitars were background music as Constance confessed the details of our upcoming test.

"Do you have to put some kind of plug in there, like a wine cork?" Jenni asked. We erupted into laughter, buzzing from the half-empty bottle of wine that had already set up camp in our blood. Constance was drinking wine only in moderation, once or twice per week, limited to one small glass, but I had given up my sobriety on Friday nights. Lyricism and melody soared and another week of thinking about and working on our infertility was diluted with every sip and every chord strummed.

"No, she's just going to check out the natural reaction, see if my body is killing Matty's sperm," Constance said.

"For all we know she could have a Yankee vagina and my sperm could be a band of Confederate soldiers. We've got to make sure there's not a war being waged over our rights to baby making, and that my sperm aren't on the losing side of the battle."

"Oh, you guys," Kamila said, hitting her bass guitar strings and sending a low moan through the living room. "That is one of the grossest things I've ever heard. I can't believe you have to do that. I'm so sorry."

Perhaps it was the bottle of wine I tanked during rehearsal or the unrelenting presence of our problem, which was now a daily issue, but that night I had a dream there were miniature AK-47s lining the insides of Constance's uterus. Smoke and debris flew through her canal as the guns popped bullets into the heads of my bandanna-covered sperm, killing them one by one before they could reach the egg. To fix the problem Dr. Leya gave me a cup of shiny silver bulletproof vests to swallow and sent me home to sleep for four months until my newly protected sperm had regained their strength.

I woke up sweating, my heart racing and my testicles receding into my body, hiding from the dangers of the destructive dream vagina. Our infertility, it seemed, was not just a daily issue; it was an around-the-clock stressor ready to pit my body against my wife's. The war, despite my passivity, was officially on.

Our drive to Evanston was brief and quiet, and as the rain began lilting from the clouds, I composed a mental list of the scores of fantastic things that have happened on stormy days. Constance and I got married, both our nieces, Aliyah and Chelsey, were born, I attended a legendary R.E.M. concert in St. Paul, Minn., and the *Cat in the Hat*, my favorite children's book, taught me as an innocent youngster, the true meaning of indoor mischief. Perhaps our postcoital exam, you see, could be as easy as one, two, three.

Dr. Leya insisted, for the first time in our budding patient-doctor relationship, that I remain in the waiting room while Constance went behind the wall for an exam. Feminism burned in my veins, boiling until the pressure behind my face and inside my head reached the precipice of the great Bruce Banner–Incredible Hulk divide. Being cut out of the process, being given orders to fork over my seed and shut up, turned me green with envy and angry with inequality. Both women who had been in the waiting room before us were now gone, so I dropped down onto the floor, ascended my body into the plank position, and began doing push-ups.

Two hundred fifty compressions and twenty minutes later, Constance emerged; her eyes were bright blue sparkling oceans, and her lips were bent upward in a satisfied grin. It was an immediate visual improvement over the last time she had emerged from the exam room, rash infested following the iodine fiasco.

"Well, what did she say?" I asked, popping up from my chair like toast on a mission.

"Everything was just fine. All of my blood work is fine, my tubes are open, and apparently I'm not killing your sperm."

"Okay, tell me more. What did she do?"

Dr. Leya swabbed Constance's vaginal mucus and put it under a microscope, counting the sperm still swimming toward freedom. Dr. Leya confirmed that the requisite number of healthy sperm were indeed present.

"Half the time I was back there was spent looking for my right ovary," Constance said. "She said the left one was up to something, but the right one wasn't, which can be normal. Both don't always prepare to release an egg every month."

"So what now?"

"We wait and see if we get pregnant this month, and if not, we do more tests. It could be that I'm ovulating too late in my cycle, or it could be nothing at all. We could be just fine, and it could just be taking a really long time. We're just going to keep trying for another month, and if that doesn't work we'll start fertility meds."

I smiled and wrapped Constance in my arms, my muscles still quivering from my angry, impromptu workout. My sperm was cleared, and I should have been relieved, but I held Constance and worried that my diet lacked enough positive nutrition to make sperm strong enough to reproduce. I didn't eat meat more than once per week, and I rarely ate fats, either good or bad. During our drive home I vowed to buy a couple of avocados and a few servings of pure animal protein to up my energy for the month's ovulation. It was something within my power to change, and I believed, despite the tests, that I still was keeping us from our baby.

Seventeen days past ovulation, seven AM on a bleary Sunday morning, and Constance still hadn't gotten her period. We had one pregnancy test on hand and decided that instead of boxing it up, tucking it between a pile of scarves and a Cuisinart as we prepared to move to a rehabbed condo two blocks from our current apartment, we'd give it a shot.

Had Constance's period not arrived in full force moments after releasing her first morning pee to the devilish stick, we would have been quite pleased with the partial second line that appeared on the test.

"What the hell does that mean?" Constance asked, holding the test up to the vanity lights. Our bathroom was empty save for a roll of toilet paper sitting on the floor and a towel hanging over the rod holding only a shower liner. "I've heard that any second line is treated like a positive result, but I know this is my period."

Constance tossed the stick back into the garbage and flushed the toilet.

"Don't throw that away. It's the closest we've gotten yet!" I said, peeling it back out of the trash and holding the dry, inconclusive test to my heart. "We're keeping this one."

Memory boxes were packed away beneath a pile of dishes and books, so I placed the test on top of the case for the *Arrested Development* DVDs next to our bedroom television. Our first second line, a one-eighth inch of significant progress, which still meant we had failed.

During my shower that morning, Constance walked into the bathroom, and without respect for my preference to soak in the radiant morning sun, flipped on the lights and said, "Please, don't say, 'Oh, Constance, why are you doing this now? Why can't you just let it go?' but I've been thinking about the paint in the condo."

My shoulders involuntarily tensed like the tightening of a screw that at any moment would become stripped and useless. I didn't want it to happen, and I began breathing in and out, readying my balloons for an early morning trip into the atmosphere. Constance's suggestion, I knew, was coming from an innocent place of outstanding style, but my reflex was to parse her challenges through a frustrated filter. Especially since this request was landing so late in the game, with only days to go before we closed on our first home, a newly constructed condo that was being outfitted to our exact specifications.

"What were you thinking of doing?" I asked, without the slightest touch of annoyance in my delivery. Bloodshed had started the day, and I forced the words out of my mouth minus the snarky tone that could have caused more to follow. Constance was bleeding and she had earned leeway for her whimsical digression.

"Well, we opted to have the second bedroom painted light gray, like the master bedroom, but when that becomes a baby room, will that be the color we want? Don't we want it the same soft green as the bathroom?"

When that becomes a baby room.

When.

She had ceased speaking in positive scenarios months ago, and without a hint of desperation or questioning, Constance spoke assuredly about parenthood for the first time since the day we purchased our condo four months previous. She stated a fact, and like any debate or argument in which my well-learned spouse engaged, I believed every word she said.

When.

"You can change it if you want, if it's not too late, but we can always paint it ourselves when the baby comes. It won't be too hard."

"If we even ever need it for a nursery," she said, ending her brief return to form, her return to the Constance of June 2006, when we were making love in the afternoon for the first time without birth control and with a hopeful vigor for our future. That woman wasn't gone, but she was reverting deeper inside of this new woman each time the cards stacked against us gained another back-breaking layer.

We officially had an infertility full deck, fifty-two weeks of letdowns, and not one winning hand.

~⁓~

"Just take off everything below the waist and put the sheet over you," Dr. Leya said on her way out the door. "I'll be right back to take a quick look for cysts, and then we'll get you a prescription for meds."

After she left, Constance began to disrobe. I took her skirt and hung it over the back of a chair to keep it wrinkle-free for our afternoon condo closing. "Well, I guess we know what our next step is," I said. "I can't believe it's come to fertility medication."

Dr. Leya returned, strapped a condom onto the end of her ultrasound wand, and coated it with lubricating jelly. Constance's wincing face and tensed upper body competed with the menacing clouds outside, which threatened to make our move even more challenging, for the most crap-tastic element of the day. Dr. Leya searched for clear views of Constance's ovaries while I stewed over the prospect of rain on our moving day, imagining dripping, heavy boxes full of our damp possessions pooling on our newly stained hardwood floors. Floors we finally owned.

Seeing my wife in pain, however, clenching her hands into fists, filled me with guilt-tinged grief. Constance's sacrifices— of her body and her sanity—to make our baby happen were paramount to a drippy move and my own inconvenience. I walked over to her, unraveled her fist, and locked her fingers into mine.

"You're doing great," I said.

"Okay, see here," Dr. Leya said, pointing to the small black-and-white screen in the upper right-hand corner of her vintage ultrasound machine. "You're clear on both sides. No cysts, so we can start you on Clomid this month. Take one pill every day for the next five days, and then come in one week from today for a shot that I will administer to you. Clomid has been around for over fifty years, and children who were conceived on Clomid are having children, so don't worry about birth defects," Dr. Leya said in her reassuring, straight-talking tone. "It does not increase your chances for triplets or quadruplets, but it does increase your chance of twins. I'm not sure why it doesn't increase your chance for triplets, since there will be more eggs available, but it doesn't."

We both knew Clomid was coming because it was always the first step for infertile couples. Every bit of research said the same thing, and we knew what Constance was in for— the mood swings, the rashes, and the intense cramping. Dr. Leya took out her prescription tablet, scribbled down the

Clomid dose on one sheet, and ripped it off.

"You guys also need to have intercourse at least every other day," she said, scribbling on a second prescription sheet. "Or every three days if that isn't possible. Do it for the next eight days to be safe. But you don't have to do it every day. You don't have to knock yourselves out," she said, handing Constance the second green sheet. "This is your prescription for sex, in case you forget. Make sure you stick to it. You can't get pregnant if you're not having sex."

Once we arrived at the elevator, Constance and I smiled at each other. "I'm in heaven. I've waited my whole life for that very prescription. I feel high."

"Much better than more pills."

"And honestly, how hard is it to have sex every other day? I can't believe she has to tell people that," I said. My libido was vigorous, but having intercourse three to four times per week seemed like a no-effort minimum.

"Most people do it once a week. They're not like us."

"Well, while I don't get that because, seriously, what else are you doing? Turn off the freakin' *C.S.I.* and get to it. But more than that, I really don't get that for couples who are trying to conceive."

"I don't get it either," Constance said. "Where's the fun in that?"

As we stepped through the electronic entrance, I grabbed Constance's butt, she grabbed mine, and we smiled in recognition of our immense luck at having each other. By then, the sun was peeking through the clouds, which had shed their darkness for a fluffy, friendly veneer. The rain was gone again, and we were ready to move and move on.

Chapter 16

· ·

Death, Love, and Crying Babies in Catholic Churches

Joe Thomas was already dead by the time Constance's period arrived on a Sunday morning in late July. Our day began as a trickle of blood, a second Clomid failure, and when Constance's cell phone rang, flashing KRISTA THOMAS in the reception window, I wanted to ignore the intrusion and go back to bed. Grieving was an essential step in my rebound process, and I wanted to collect my one day without interruption or contact with the outside world that didn't care about my sadness and move toward a prosperous next chance.

"I should answer it, Matty," she said. "Krista usually only calls when it's something important."

Two hours later, every inch of our new granite countertop was blanketed by combination of sugar and butter. Peanut butter cup brownies, banana bars, chocolate chip cookies, and peanut butter cookies stacked on plain white plates easily could have been a reaction to losing our July baby. However, on this particular Sunday, another babyless month destined to be shuffled and lost in the deck, our excessive baking was the only way to avoid succumbing to the numbness we felt after hearing the news about Joe.

Joe was Krista's twenty-three-year-old little brother, her lone sibling, and it took just one early morning drive on the Eden's Expressway and just one egregious driver error to erase the verve of Constance's best friend in Chicago.

Joe was a big guy, an ex-college football player and long-time lothario, and I dug having him around because he was one in only a handful of people that made me feel small in stature. He adored his sister, and I was often taken by his reverence for her, by his sly, confident gaze that reminded me of a cross between Joey from *Friends* and a smarter looking Nick Carter from the Backstreet Boys. Joe treated Krista with dignity, respect, and little-brother hero worship. My admiration for Joe was based primarily on his skill for loving one of my favorite people in the world.

After Constance hung up the phone, we sat motionless on the sofa for fifteen minutes and said nothing as the "Sports Reporters" continued debating the headlines of the week in spite of their insignificance.

"What do we do?" Constance asked. "This is so awful. Joe and Gina just got engaged, and the whole family was so excited. What do you think we should do for her? Krista is one of my best friends and I want to be there for her, but she grew up here. She'll have so many people around her right now who've known her longer, but I have to do something. I can't do nothing for her. Krista wouldn't do nothing."

Parents are made for such moments, and mine, I knew, would give me the answer and the calm I sought. I wanted to hear their voices, to tell them how Krista's life had changed forever and how happy I was to be alive and still have the luxury of calling them on a Sunday morning. And, as if I was once again twelve years old and deciding between following my talents toward music or a more socially acceptable endeavor such as football, I wanted them to tell me what to do.

"Well, here in Iowa we make food," Mom said. "When somebody dies, we bake a bunch of casseroles and desserts for the family because they aren't going to feel like cooking or even thinking about food."

"Cookies and brownies are always good comfort foods," Dad said. "Plus, they'll have so many people coming and going it will be good to have portable stuff for people to take. Sad people like sugar. Or maybe that's just me."

I didn't know Joe that well. We met for the first time at a fundraiser at T's bar in Andersonville and had on several occasions thereafter bonded via tequila shots at parties thrown by Krista and Cheryl. But it would have been spitting in the face of fortune not to feel grateful that morning and not to call my parents and tell them how lucky I was to have them in my life.

"I love you guys," I said as my throat constricted and my mind flooded with the always present worry that I would be too far away when the inevitable happened in my own family.

"You're a good boy, Matthew," Mom said. "Your dad and I love you so much. You guys just be safe today, okay. We worry about you all of the time."

Krista's family was now reduced to a mother and a father and a sister grasping to understand how their delicately balanced table would remain steady upon three legs. My table was still five-legs strong, and I wanted to sit myself around it and never move again because I knew that no table remains unwobbly forever.

"We baked until we ran out of sugar," Constance said as we unpacked six grocery bags full of sweets, ten paper plates, stacking them on the bare Formica countertops and, once space ran out, onto the blackened gas stovetop.

"We didn't know what else to do," I said, "and we had to do something, so we thought we'd keep going until we couldn't go any more. The sugar was the first to go."

"Butter wasn't far behind," Constance said. Krista, Cheryl, and their friend Rachel had just come back from picking up Joe's Chevy Tahoe from the parking lot where he had parked it before getting into someone else's car. Unexpected laughter crawled out of their mouths as tears still scarred their eyes.

"You guys are so crazy," Krista said, bending her six-foot frame down to embrace Constance. "There's enough sugar here to send us into a coma."

Everyone in the room was talking about details of what had happened, what was to come, and what needed to be done to draw a straight line between the two obstacles. A reporter from the *Sun Times* called, the third reporter of the day, and Krista's anger at having to give a statement about how the family was feeling sent her into a rage of tears and rightful condescension. "My brother's dead; how do you think I feel? I feel awful," she said, slamming the phone and sobbing onto Cheryl's shoulder. "I wish they would stop. Would you believe a TV reporter showed up at our doorstep at, like, seven this morning?"

Standing in the shadow of Krista's grief and that of her mother, still clothed in her white cloth nightgown, inconsolable and near collapse, I was flooded with an urgent surge, a need to do whatever it took to get a family of my own. Intense love and the connection that adheres to any flavor of family unit, biological or otherwise, is the most challenging and rewarding bond to achieve. Krista's family had loved and lost, had been pummeled by a barrage of uppercuts and jabs, grieving at having lost out on the future they didn't see coming. Joe's loss and the torture that ensued only served to illuminate how rewarding and important it is to achieve what we had failed.

Family is everything and nobody is better off without it.

Joe's funeral was a wholly Catholic affair. Polish Catholic to be exact, which led to an hour and a half of standing, kneeling, sitting, praying, and sobbing. All of which was closely followed by countless rounds of food and beverages served up by white-and-black-clad waiters in a Polish banquet hall. Sausages, sauerkraut, pierogies, liver and dumplings, chicken, and beef were all served as a gut-busting tribute to our dear friend's brother.

Churches had always made me fidgety, even under the best of circumstances. I was in a house of God that was not my home. The stress of the funeral coupled with my inherent unease saw me hugging the people in the pews around me when we were merely called upon to shake hands, which was the first of many mistakes I made in violation of the unspoken religious law.

"I'm sorry, I'm not very good at this," I said to Deirdre, a friend of Krista's who was seated next to us. "I don't really know what I'm doing. If I slip up just tell me what to do. Sometimes when I'm at a church service I feel like a virgin fumbling with a bra strap."

"Me, too," Deirdre said, "although not with a bra strap. Maybe a zipper. But I totally get ya. And I even went to Catholic school. My grandmother would be so disappointed."

Two pews in front of us, a young woman was struggling to

contain the pacifier and slightly jarring coos of a less-than-
two-year-old toddler as Gina's mom stoically revealed the
irreparable heartbreak of her daughter, who had purchased her
wedding dress the day before the accident. The toddler was a
perfect, dark-skinned, dark-eyed beauty with a mat of curls
secured on the top of her head by a small pink bow. Her tone-
shifting fits of laughter, in contrast to the raw eulogy of a dev-
astated mother, unnerved me. I couldn't help but conjecture
that a child was out of place at such a silent mourning, that her
laughter clashed with the oppressive sadness.

If that was my kid, I wouldn't just sit there, I thought,
wishful that the slightly plump mother would gather her
cartoon-emblazoned diaper bag and blankets and step out
into the hallway and give us all a reprieve from any hint of
happiness. But the moment our eyes met, the baby girl's
jovial brown button eyes oblivious to the talk of Joe's plush
room in heaven, her grin froze my gaze and blocked out the
priest's oratory. The unease that his reverent words had
caused in my stomach immediately blended into the background of creaking pews and shifting people, and instead of
fear and sadness, I was overcome by a sense of strength.
Suddenly she seemed to be the only one that belonged in a
house of worship.

I wanted to believe that she was staring at me, that her joy
was derived from the joy I deflected back to her, but Constance,
Deirdre, and at least seven other warm bodies in the vicinity

were also garnering affection and power from this noisy, cheery little Smurf. Church finally made sense to me in the presence of this baby and this acknowledgement of Joe's passing, and remembrance of his legacy became not about God or death or sadness, but about love.

Life in its purest form can never be contained, and the effect we have on others is immense and often unintended. Joe was laid to rest, Constance began her second round of Clomid, and that little girl probably went home to watch today's TiVoed episode of *Sesame Street* and massage a bowl of cold cereal into her flaxen curls. Nothing ever really ends, nothing ever really stops—even when pieces of you die or you find yourself unable to get pregnant or live your life without your brother.

Somehow people keep on finding new ways to exist that honor the remnants and revisions of life, letting go of a vision that never really existed in the first place to embrace a world they didn't want.

Constance and my final picture wouldn't be a Van Gogh because that was an idealistic picture I painted in my head that had no basis in reality. After a string of anything's possible years, our plan for a perfect life of master's degrees, a stylish home, and two children felt attainable, but I now knew that not everything would be easy and not everything should be. As long as our picture rose above the insipid pandering of a Thomas Kincade landscape, I was willing to work harder for something I truly wanted. Losing two hundred and sixty pounds was proof that I could run a thousand circles for one chance at a straight line to the finish.

Joe's legacy, for me, was a reminder that the straight line existed and that it was my responsibility to run as fast as possible until I found it.

Chapter 17

· ·

The Fast, the Furious, and an
Iris Through the Looking Glass

August felt unfamiliar as we limped into another month, our fourteenth, without so much as a late period to ebb or tide our hopes. A literal limp had also become part of my life; my feet no longer could fly across the concrete to relieve the stress of our infertility via exertion. One leg brace banned me from the rapid life due to a severe case of tendonitis in my left foot, and my overall mood had shifted from petulant to insufferable.

"So what do you do for a living?" Dr. Amaranth asked, contorting my ailing paw into painful pose after painful pose. Each bend was a shock vibrating from the center of my flat foot into the anterior tibial tendon running from the side of my foot up the inside of my leg. I had begun to experience pain during my first USTA league tennis match in Grant Park, and the severity worsened as I sprinted boxes up and down a flight of stairs moving into our new condo.

After our fourth night of moving and unloading, we ran to Whole Foods for some ice cream, and I could barely walk myself back to the car, at which time I negotiated an agreement with Constance: one pint of Ben & Jerry's Primary Berry ice cream all to myself in exchange for one immediate date with the foot specialist. By August I finally made good on my word.

"I'm a writer and the creative Web director for a newspaper syndicate," I said to the doctor, rolling my eyes in preparation for the inevitable. I knew better than to be honest and regretted not stowing away the nature of my work, burying it alongside the pain he was purposely prolonging by modeling my foot in every imaginable pose. Unprepared to divulge the nature and scope of my job, I just wanted to get my foot fixed and go home. I wanted to take off running from his office and never return, but each step made me queasy and a major component of being an effective nonfiction writer was being open and honest, so I told him about my health and fitness writing. "And I write a syndicated blog," I said, dovetailing my words in hopes he would be too preoccupied staging my extremity to fully understand.

"That's outstanding," he said, dropping my foot to the floor and extending his hand. I exchanged my hand for my foot and he shook it heartily. "What's your blog about?" I gave him the canned answer—nothing too risqué or insightful but enough to build a wall that hopefully he could not jump or tear down.

"Oh, that's a really noble, ripe topic," he said. "You know, when my wife and I were trying to conceive our second child, about six months into the process we had gotten nowhere. When I came home one day there were stacks of books about how to solve your infertility problems strewn about the living room. Thankfully we got pregnant the next month or I would have had to actually read all of those tomes."

"Yeah, I haven't really taken the self-help plunge, yet," I said, "but it has been a rough go. The greatest part of it all is writing this story and finding out there are so many people just like me. The older I get the more I take comfort in the fact that I'm insignificant. When I was younger I wanted to believe that I was totally unique and nobody on Earth experienced the world like I did. Now, that seems like a burden, and I relish the fact that there are countless people just like me."

"It took me until I was forty to realize that," Dr. Amaranth said. "And you know, is there anything in the world that's more fun to practice until you get it right? Especially now that you can't run or play tennis?"

"Yeah, it is for me, anyway, right now. But not for everybody. Sex isn't as fun when you're angry at the world."

"I'm sure even running would get tiresome if you never got anywhere," he said.

As it turned out my tendon was neither torn nor ruptured. And Dr. Amaranth was just another man with another story and a slightly inappropriate take on our fourteenth-month-

and-counting attempt to conceive. Only his story didn't strike me as funny, and his brief six-month struggle struck me as a being nothing more than a dead fly making his final resting place on a radar screen with thousands of non-stop flights.

When Katie, my physical therapist in Andersonville, asked the most unnecessary of questions, "So, are you ready to run?" I barely could wipe the remnants of the cold blue ultrasound gel from my ankle before I was upright on the treadmill for the first time in nearly eight weeks. Treadmills are one of those design oddities, much like the futon, that inherently blends functionality with ugliness and pain, and both have made an unfortunate impact in living rooms across the world. As much as I loved running, on the flip side of that emotional high is my disdain for electronic movement. After two months, however, I was ready to kiss the moving belt on which I walked, and subsequently began to run.

Going nowhere, staring out the window at the green trees and blue sky peering over the top of the mattress store along Clark Street, I saw a girl, roughly four years old, all curls and big eyes, standing with her bald, middle-aged father waiting for a north-bound bus. At first she was reticent to catch my eye or approach the glass, but as she winked at me and I winked in return, she began to shift her feet like an old man dancing, shuffling toward the window to get a better view of the fascinating man and his running machine.

I cocked my head sideways, first to the left and then to the right, and began to tick my head like the pendulum of a clock that had all the time in the world. Her face lit up, and she ran toward the window and began to bounce up and down on the balls of her pink-sandaled feet. Her father, once he noticed her absence, briskly came up behind her and swooped her back to the bus stop.

They stood next to the bus stop sign, gazing down the street in anticipation of its arrival, but it wasn't one minute before I caught her gaze again and began to play peek-a-boo while dashing at a seven-mile-per-hour clip. She jogged to the window again and took her turn in our eye-hiding game. Sweat was bubbling to the surface of my forehead, and the little girl in front of me popped from side to side, jumping up and down and giggling as I stuck my tongue out and pretended to struggle to keep pace with the treadmill.

By this time her father had arrived at her side and I gave him the "okay signal," and he laughed along with us. The man was about fifty pounds overweight and a little sloppy in his baggy business shirt and ill-fitting cargo pants. When he looked at me, he patted his bulbous tummy and nodded his head, then pointed at me and gave a thumbs-up. He told me, without a word, to keep up the good work in my fitness.

I looked at him, pointed at his daughter, and gave him a

thumbs-up in return, and without a word told him to keep up the good work with his child. He smiled, picked up his daughter, and carried her back to the stop, where they boarded the waiting bus and then disappeared into the city.

A buzzer rang in the background, and Katie shouted across the packed workout space that my fifteen minutes were up— the fifteen minutes I had waited all summer to experience. Pushing the button to slow the treadmill to three miles per hour, I walked for five minutes to cool my muscles, toweling my sweat off of the bars and control panel. Pain never emerged from my foot and I was covered in a thin veneer of sweat, but I remembered nothing about the actual foot-after-foot run from which I had been in withdrawal. I did, however, remember I was still running in place toward something that's just on the other side of the looking glass.

That day, however, for the first time, it looked back at me and smiled in the middle of the race.

Chapter 18

· ·

More Death, More Love, and More than Words

Driving along the flat and lifeless stretch of I–80 was both visually and mentally stunting on its own accord without the addition of broken A/C in the PT Cruiser. Two days earlier my parents called with the news that Aunt Ruth had died from complications during her hip surgery.

Constance and I stewed over the flows of hot, recycled air puffing through the vents for hours on end. I plucked disintegrating ice cubes from a Subway cup to curb Marcy's steady panting that consumed the stale oxygen in our cabin. Topping it all off, Constance's preovulation cramps began to escalate in tandem with the temperature.

"Let's take personality quizzes on your iPhone to pass the time," Constance suggested. Content That Works, the newspaper syndicate where I work and play, had recently supplied all employees with a free iPhone and complimentary service, and since that time my life had been infused with a bit of rock star.

"I hope someday Steve Jobs will take the stage to celebrate the launch of the highly anticipated iBaby, and then all infertiles can dispose of the Clomid supply, cancel the IVF treatments, and collect our technologically flawless children capable of storing 15,000 songs for the reasonable price of five hundred ninety-nine dollars," I said, surfing the Web as we made the long trip back to Chicago.

"Well, I guess it will at least help us pass the time," Constance said, fanning her hand in front of her face. I grabbed an ice cube from the cup and rubbed it across the back of her neck. "God, that feels so good. I wish you could rub that all over my body." Instead of fulfilling her fantasy and mine—pulling the car to the side of the road, disrobing, and covering ourselves in ice cubes—we took quiz after quiz, answering questions about everything from ice cream preference to how to cross a river. Every test returned the same results: Constance prioritizes her life with money first and family second, and I am the most important person in her life. I was family first and money second.

"Do you think we'll ever have a baby?" Constance asked as traffic slowed as we neared the outlet malls in Aurora marking our arrival to the Chicago area.

"I definitely do," I said.

It had been a tough weekend on the stick-in-the-eye front. During the dinner following Aunt Ruth's funeral, my cousin Cody announced that his wife was pregnant—with their second child since we had begun trying to conceive our first.

"So when's it your turn?" my childhood friend, Rachel, asked Constance while holding our niece Aliyah. It was hard not to feel nonparental claustrophobia while holding court in the new Lutheran church on the outskirts of Winterset, eating warm macaroni salad, and offering quick snippets of your life to people who no longer know much about you.

"We're trying," I said, draping my arm around Constance's shoulders. "It's just not happening very easily."

"I don't know, Matthew," Cody said. "You just might want to stick with dogs."

"Yeah, I love my dog," I said, standing up from the family table and moving toward the unappetizing buffet line.

We drove back to Chicago that night, trekking seven hours across two states in order to make our appointment with Dr. Leya the next morning. Constance had already taken the third round of Clomid pills and was now ready for the painful stab in the ass that would engage ovulation.

"You've got three eggs that are all contenders," Dr. Leya said. "Your ovaries look good and healthy. Now I want you guys to have sex today, tomorrow, and the next day just to be safe. Here's your sex prescription for the next three days. If you don't have your period in fourteen days, take a test and come into the office."

This is a giant waste of time, I thought. *Something more is wrong and we just don't know it. Clomid is not the answer for us.* Thoughts of self-blame were once again knocking at the door, and instead of waiting to see if the big bad wolf could blow the house down, I just wanted to make him a spare set of keys and get it over with. I craved bad news. An unexplained diagnosis left me nothing to work on and nothing to dwell on, and so I had no choice but to take it out on myself.

This is all my fault.

"Let's get a second dog," I said on the drive home. "Let's go this weekend."

By Monday, Grace had contacted me with word that she was eager to take me on as a client: the paperwork was in the mail, and beyond that, she already had a publisher interested in my work. After three years of searching for an agent to take on my weight loss memoir, shopping it to agents and publishers up and down the coasts, I had found someone to represent me in less than one week thanks to Bev, a freelancer I worked with who had taken an interest in my blog. Only it wasn't for the completed manuscript about my former obesity; rather, a book about our infertility.

"The time is ripe for an idea like this," Grace said through the phone, as I sat in the lobby of the Chrysler dealership, getting the air conditioner hose repaired that had engendered our road trip misery. Maria, the woman behind the counter who had given me a wink as she ushered me to my seat, was staring at my exaggerated happiness. Something good had finally come of all of this, and I was finally filled with a sense of purpose, a way to make reason out of what had happened. "How soon can you get me a sample?"

"I suppose by next Friday," I said, emphatically tapping my right foot against the floor like a heavy metal drummer at his kit. Major portions of my joy were derived from finally achieving my goals, but I was almost equally thrilled to be working on a sample that didn't involve my right hand, a plastic cup, and a hospital lavatory.

On the drive home, I chose to disobey Illinois traffic laws and drove with only one hand on the wheel as I began to work my way through contact after contact, my mom, sister, best friends, and colleagues, to share my news. I quickly discovered that for infertile folk like myself, the phrase "So, I have some great news" is off-limits and should be banned from the infertile vocabulary until procreation is successful.

"You're pregnant?" my friend Sarah queried.

"No, we're not pregnant," I said, unsure how to slyly unwrap her pristine gift of elation and still give her back something equally compelling in an unadorned paper bag. If babies are toys from Santa on Christmas morning, then success surely is a package of underwear from Grandma the night before.

Calls to my bandmates, Kamila and Jenni, elicited the same response.

I began to temper every call with "So, we're not pregnant,

but I have some really great news." It was the ski-slope approach of delivering my message—slowly driving my loved ones up the hill, dropping them off the cliff, and starting all over again, hoping the second trip down the mountain would be nearly as exciting as the first.

For the first time I felt the twinge, the grumblings in my belly, of being consumed by an inorganic process. The new Tori Amos album thumped through the speakers of the car stereo as I sat outside our apartment and began the march toward signing off with my sister April. Fall was falling everywhere I turned, and from my perch in the driver's seat, clutching a Venti coffee in one hand and an iPhone to my ear, it was impossible to escape the changing of the guard currently storming the gates in the form of yellow and orange leaves.

Fall had come again and we were still crouched down, hands to the ground at the starting gates, waiting for a gunshot and some momentum. Sex was easy and getting pregnant was a right of passage that was passing us by with its middle fingers hoisted into the air.

"Yeah, it's really exciting," I said, unsure if my response was appropriate to the words April had ceased speaking because I had lost my thoughts and hers in the changing trees. "I love you, April."

"I love you too, Matty," she said. "I'm very proud of you."

Brian from across the hall walked by the car and gave me a conservative wave, dipping down to make sure I wasn't having some sort of diabetic episode or seizure, as I sat with my forehead against the steering wheel and the music at full tilt. I smiled and waved him on, holding my phone up hoping to send the message that I was waiting for a call instead of the return of my sanity. After hanging up with April, I needed a moment of nothing but loud music and head banging before heading upstairs to take Marcy and our new shepherd mix puppy, Hazel, for a walk.

After the song ended, I exited the car and grabbed the mail. Two more envelopes from our insurance company sandwiched Senator Fred Thompson's rickety frame on the cover of *Newsweek*. Since beginning treatments with Dr. Leya, we had consumed two hundred dollar ultrasounds like rappers in jewelry boutiques dropping limitless dough on yellow diamonds. Inexplicably expensive blood tests and injectibles were not a concern, because Blue Cross Blue Shield of Illinois would send us frivolous "This is not a bill" notifications and any inkling of financial burden was instantly deleted from our minds.

"Two more 'This is not a bill' statements from the insurance company," I said, handing the mail to Constance, her daily gift of task satisfaction, and kissing her smooth forehead. "I wish there was some way we could tell them to stop sending us those. We've gotten enough to wallpaper this whole condo in 'this is not a bill' notices. Not that anybody would want to do that, but you know what I mean. It's a waste."

"What the hell? It says we owe three hundred sixty-eight

dollars, Matty," Constance said, shoving the piece of paper into my face.

"Too close, too close! Make Matty go blind," I said, pushing her hands out of my face into a comfortable reading distance. "Holy crap, this is a bill. Oh, man. That's so much money."

"I guess we finally exceeded our limit for the year," Constance said. "We're really going to have to start being frugal with money. We can't afford these kinds of bills and the expensive Whole Foods bills, and all of the eating out and going to movies and concerts."

What had been a free packet of seeds had blossomed into a nearly four-hundred-dollar weed that threatened to overtake our financial garden and kill every blooming flower.

"Paying for this is going to suck," I said. "It's not like we're guaranteed anything cool, like an iPod or a trip to Wimbledon on the flipside. We keep paying to have wands shoved in your hoo-ha, for me to masturbate at the hospital, and for us to be criminally disappointed every month."

"Yeah, hopefully it won't be too much of a burden. It looks like they didn't cover one of my tests for some reason. We'll just have to start saving more in the service of Baby. And then we'll make Baby pay us back once he or she is a tennis prodigy."

"What sucks is I know we need to save money now, but why then do I want a pizza?"

"Because, it's coming," she said. "I feel really PMSy."

I said nothing in return, not because I was sad or upset

about the possibility that this round of Clomid, our fourth, wasn't going to work, but because I was still thinking about the pizza and knew we no longer had the luxury of ordering it.

"I'm making macaroni and cheese," I said. "If I can't have pizza, I need something that will make me feel really gross and happy."

After our cheesy lunch, we sat on the sofa to watch a Food Network cake challenge, and Constance leaned into me. Her hair smelled like it used to when we were dating, with overtones of flowers and sex.

"I'm sorry I let you down," she said, pushing her face into my chest and shaking her head.

"How in the world could you possibly have let me down?"

"Well, if this is PMS, then I'm not pregnant again."

"That doesn't let me down at all," I said. "You have never let me down. And we don't really know yet. And even if it is your period, that just means another month of just the two of us. And I'll always welcome more time with my baby."

Instead of sitting around and dreaming of food until we justified ordering a pizza, and instead of getting ahead of ourselves in terms of the PMS, the symptoms that could or could not signal another failed month, we went bowling and played pinball in Lincoln Square, spending money we didn't have to keep ourselves safe from the vivid imaginations we had. And there we proved to each other and to the world that while we are terrible bowlers and less-than-capable pinball wizards, we, the couple, could operate just fine with or without a pizza or a pregnancy.

~————~

"Wait, that's an ovulation test," I said, grabbing the plastic covered stick out of Constance's hand. PMS symptoms aside, the day for testing set out by Dr. Leya had arrived with no blood in sight. "I don't even think we have any pregnancy tests in the house. It's been a seriously long time since we've needed one."

"I could have sworn we had one, but I guess I just assumed these ovulation tests were pregnancy tests," Constance said. "Not like it matters. I know my period is coming. I can just feel it."

"Well, you could just go ahead and use the ovulation test," I said. "We'll probably get the same results either way. But if you want, I wouldn't mind going to the pharmacy to buy one anyway. Just to celebrate the fact that we made it to the right day, at least."

We leashed the two dogs and made the four-block trip down Ainslie and Damen and dropped twenty dollars on three tests and went home to produce just one more line.

Chapter 19

. . . .

Turkeys, Cancer, and
Alfred's Only Eye

"They ate Alfred!" Constance shouted. I pulled her shrill shriek away from my ear and leaned into the painted wood heads that served as the seat back for our office picnic table. "The puppies ate Alfred's face and nose! He's ruined."

It was a brisk Friday morning five weeks prior to Thanksgiving. Constance and I completed our first dose of October's sex prescription that morning, and I was in a postsex haze, staring at my computer and typing nothing that adhered to the rules of AP Style and no words of multiple syllables.

Unable to rebound and write my morning blog post, I solicited my friend Orion to grab coffees from the local Starbucks with me and discuss a behavioral matter involving his son.

By the time I returned to the office, having helped my friend digest his problems, I was bombarded by two problems of my own.

"You are a wanted man," Aja, our office manager, said. "Constance called and didn't sound too good, and then your mother-in-law called and said there's an urgent family matter."

An f-bomb dropped from my lips, a rarity in the workplace, and exploded in the ears of every coworker in the vicinity. Susan had told us earlier in the week her test results would arrive on Friday, and I knew the mystery behind the urgent family matter in question before I grabbed my cell phone and called Susan to confirm.

When Constance was sobbing, I assumed her mother was the basis of her grief. Unfortunately, she had yet to learn of the truly bad news of the day.

Alfred was Constance's childhood stuffed bear, and Alfred was the one thing she has always promised to grab on the way out the door in case of fire. Sometimes I felt jealous of her devotion for Alfred. If it were between him and me, I'm not so sure my fierce blue eyes and bald head could stand up to his beady black gaze and fuzzy body.

And our puppies ate his face off on the very day she was to find out her mom had cancer again. It was beginning to feel like a landslide.

"Is there anything we can do to save or fix Alfred?" I asked.

"Not unless they poop out his eyes and nose," she sobbed. I didn't mean to, but as humorous reflexes often go, I started laughing at an inappropriate time. I called with the expectation of consoling my grieving wife about her mother's illness, and instead I was dealing with an appetizer of childhood trauma.

I left the office, and five minutes later, I stood in the hallway of our condo and held my shivering wife, who shielded Alfred inside of her zipped-up hooded sweatshirt, as she sobbed for the childhood in crisis.

"Baby, I'm sorry, but I'm afraid I have even worse news," I said. "Your mom's cancer is back."

We had the dubious honor of celebrating two Thanksgivings that year to appease both wings of our family. The first was spent in North Carolina six days before the actual holiday, defrosting and feasting on an out-of-the box meal—smoked turkey, cranberries, stuffing, and potatoes, all encrusted with a thin sheen of ice that slowly pooled in the center of eight plastic containers. A holiday on thin ice, with an ill mother-in-law, two disheartened and infertile children, and a deathly family dog whose fur had begun to fall out in quarter-size crop circles. All of us feasted on the carbohydrates and simple sugars, hour after hour, in an attempt to fill the cracks in our pain with food.

Our second Thanksgiving, celebrated on the traditional day, was spent languishing in the basement of the Peru United Methodist Church, freebasing sugar in myriad forms and trying not to be petty enough, in the local house of God, to complain about arid turkey and stuffing edible only with a spoon. That also was the day I stood in the window of my childhood bedroom, postcoital, and searched the Peru landscape for a sign as to why our baby had yet to come.

Both celebrations, separated by thousands of miles but united by thousands of empty calories, were marred by our infertility. First the arrival of Constance's period, and then the prospect of our first insemination, the first domino that shoved a snaking trail of dominoes into collapse and in an unwanted direction toward a wanted pregnancy.

Insemination. I couldn't conjure the courage necessary to unveil our plan, or utter the word, to our parents, especially now that Susan's cancer had returned. Pumpkin pie in hand, fueled by an after-dinner carbohydrate rush, I should have told my in-laws, "So, your daughter is going to be inseminated in two weeks." But the proof is in the utterance, and we had yet to say the words to ourselves, and with the onslaught of family darting unannounced in and out of rooms, privacy was at a premium.

Insemination and Thanksgiving don't mix beyond the trite jokes about turkey basters, and I wanted no part of attempts to lighten the mood via inappropriate turkey humor.

Susan's colon cancer had returned, discovered four weeks prior to our trip, and our arrival in Pinehurst for holiday number one marked a time for us to make decisions regarding her care. First morning light poked at my eyes through the plantation shutters, and with Susan tucked in her bed for at least another hour, our needs for intimacy momentarily superseded the holiday spirit or planning her cancer treatments.

From her distant twin bed, a gulf not even my orangutan arms could bridge, Constance announced her period was still a no-show.

"I'm open for business," she joked. "I'm so glad we can have sex again." Clomid stuck her with yet another yeast infection, and following her fertile period, our coital habits were placed on a two-week hiatus. "Just let me go to the bathroom quickly."

I grabbed *A Thousand Splendid Suns* from the night stand, a harrowing Afghanistan war tale, which stood in stark contrast to my expanding desires, and bolted from my twin bed, trailing my wife in search of multitasked mental and physical stimulation.

Constance's period arrived before I could settle on which folded page that marked my spot.

"I guess I'm going to shower now," Constance said, flashing me the blood stained two-ply before flushing what could have been something down the toilet.

"Yeah, okay," I said. "I'm going to go back to bed and read my book." Afghanistan or Pinehurst, loss of life or loss of hope, bloodshed to bloodshed, the world felt inescapably bad, and it all occurred before my first cup of coffee.

~⌒~

"You just need to do what my doctor told me," ninety-five-year-old Aunt Bea said. "Take your temperature every day, and when it gets all hot up in there, then you have the intercourse." Constance's Aunt Bea once asked us how they taught that duck on television to talk and sell insurance. This was another beautifully awkward moment in Aunt Bea lore heard vibrantly through the crackling cell phone.

"Did Aunt Bea have infertility issues?" I asked. "I didn't know anyone in your family did."

Constance's deep, chesty chuckle, in decrescendo, faded to a hum as she wrapped her arms around my waist and playfully tugged the top of my jeans.

"Aunt Bea never had kids," she said. "I'm not sure why she didn't, but I guess it sounds like maybe she did have something wrong."

"Maybe it was before the time of diagnostics," I said. "Probably well before Clomid." Aside from my sister Angie, whom had over half of her cervix removed to ward off future cancers, there was no branch in either family tree that we could shake to find a hidden cause.

Richard and Susan's Christmas tree stood in front of the French doors that open onto the screened-in porch. Reflected in the glass, two trees, one merely a ghost, lit the gracious living room. I sat on the sofa reading my book with Riley resting his brittle canine head on my lap. He moved like an animated Japanese ghost, marching on the hardwood floors in slow, choppy movements. I tried to dig into my novel while the rest of the family watched a movie, to escape once again to Afghanistan, but my own ghost was not as docile as those of an early Christmas or a dying dog.

I put down my book on the coffee table and shifted Riley's head onto Susan's knee. Constance was on the floor, snuggled under a quilt, and I wanted to hold her, to wrap my arms around her, close my eyes and press my face into her breasts. Squeezing Constance, sometimes squeezing her forcefully enough to elicit a playful groan, was the greatest way to relieve physical stress. I had been holding her for only a moment before Sandra Bullock kissed her beau, the melodramatic score soared, and the credits rolled.

When I looked up at Susan, her body was sunk into the seams of the brown leather sofa and her eyes were bleeding tears.

"Mom, what's wrong?" Constance asked. "Is everything okay?"

Susan's sadness is as infectious as a laugh or a beat-heavy pop song, designed to make you feel and move whether you want to or not. Sometimes overbearing, demanding, and prone to bellowing your name like an unending siren until you acquiesce and cower to her every desire in lieu of matricide, Susan can be as difficult as she is loving. But when Susan is sad everyone suffers the wound because she is, more than anything, generous and pure.

"I'm just scared," she said. "Thinking about cancer is just really hard right now." Constance and I rose up from our faux floor bed and walked to the sofa to hold her. "Having you kids here is such a comfort. It's like a steaming cup of tea on a cold, rainy day when the leaves are falling from the trees."

"Mom, I love you, but you're so weird."

"What? I think that's nice."

"I think you're nice," I said, kissing the side of her warm, red face. "But not as nice as that pumpkin pie. Anybody want some more?"

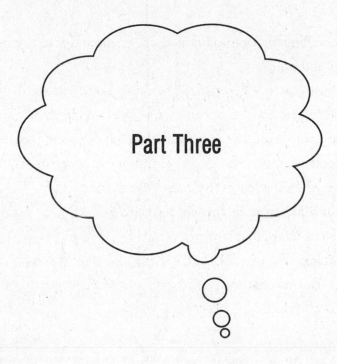

Part Three

Sex Doesn't Make Babies,
Doctors Do

Chapter 20

• •

IUI, Genauseau, and the Pine Valley Dilemma

The six-foot long orange and gray scarf was double looped around my neck like a warm winter noose. Each step toward the electronic entrance of Resurrection Hospital caused the wool fibers to catch and tug the hairs along the underside of my jaw. I tied the knot tight enough to keep the cold from penetrating my body on a frigid day in which penetration would not be necessary. We had hung from the fertility rafters for too long, swinging from sex to pills to shots, and Constance and I were finally breathless and ready to cut the cord. It was time to remove sex from the reproduction equation. On the last day in November, parked in the last row of the hospital parking lot, we stilled ourselves in the cool car seats before we tried the last thing we ever expected would be necessary to get us pregnant: artificial insemination.

Torn muscles in my right forearm, an injury achieved by single-handedly pulling a drum kit up a lengthy staircase, dictated that I use a partial cast. For this particular morning, however, I made an exception and instead wrapped the gauze around the molded image of my arm and tucked it inside my koi fish-embroidered satchel.

"You need to keep wearing that, Matty," Constance said. "Your arm won't get better if you don't start wearing it more."

"I'm not going to bother putting the cast on now," I said. "I know I'm not going to be able to masturbate with my left hand. That hand is pretty much dead to me—a nonentity."

Masturbating left-handed isn't impossible, and I knew from experience I could bring myself to climax ambidextrously. Directing my semen sample into the small lab cup, left-handed, however, while crouched, pants gathered around my ankles in a single-stall bathroom, would not be an easy feat. And no amount of pain in my forearm or psyche would be worth making a mistake and ruining our first insemination attempt.

"Won't that hurt you?" Constance asked.

"Probably," I said impatiently, "but I'd rather have my dominant hand at the ready because I'm not really excited about jerking off in the hospital bathroom again, and I don't have a lot of time to finish."

Patronizing my second hospital restroom, situating myself for the third time in the epicenter of cacophonous medical diagnostics to make sexy time with myself in the unsexiest of settings was not a moment I wanted to linger. Pleasure had become more complicated than achieving an erection and bringing myself to climax. Such findings, nuggets of infertility wisdom collected throughout the last sixteen months, were beginning to further distance me from my youth. Emerging gray chin hairs were now more than an early unfortunate sign of aging—they were symbolic of an adult journey full of adult decisions and a foreseeable future of unenjoyable masturbation—unfathomable less than nine months ago, the first time I gave an in-hospital semen sample. But a lot can happen—and an even greater lot cannot happen—in nine months.

At our appointment the previous morning, we quietly sat in uncomfortable chairs in Dr. Leya's modest, topsy-turvy office, loose papers and files decorating every available surface, the walls entirely bare save for two framed diplomas and a handful of licenses. "So, here's your sample cup," she said. "Now, you can either do the sample in the lab or do it at home. That's up to you. If you do it at home, Constance, you'll need to put the cup with the sample in your bra on the way to the hospital tomorrow. It's too cold outside."

"I guess that makes sense," Constance said. "So, I need to keep it warm?"

"Not warm, but about room temperature," she said. "Just keep it in your bra, and that will be perfect." Dr. Leya looked up at me, a four-inch smile cutting across my face as visions of Constance tucking my semen sample into her bra began to blossom in my head like deformed flowers in a Dr. Seuss book. Dignity had never been a priority for me, and even then, as the endocrinologist conductor shouted, "Last call!" for the express brassiere train for which my semen now held a one-way ticket, it was not a matter of pride or embarrassment. Moment upon moment of bizarre requests, conversations, and procedures had finally merged into one super, Voltron-like being that was even too weird for me.

Dr. Leya instructed us to arrive at the lab no later than seven AM the next day—insemination day.

I couldn't let our maybe baby be transported to the hospital via Constance's chest. The line finally had been crossed, and instead of a tear or a burst of anger, I allowed myself to laugh the entire trip home.

"Wow, you know, every time we go there it's something unexpected," Constance said as we approached the elevator. Nobody ever occupied the circuitous, square hallway, which provided us a private place to decompress following our visits. "I would never in a million years have imagined that I'd one day carry your semen in my bra to a hospital so a doctor could inseminate me."

"I'm just going to do the sample at the lab," I said on the walk back to the car. "I am not going to make you carry my semen in your bra. I just won't do it." Participatory demands on me had become few and far between following my initial semen analysis. Constance took the mood-altering pills, the shots in the butt and the twice-monthly ultrasounds. No matter how much I wanted to masturbate in the comfort of my own home, I could not ask her to drive the six miles to the hospital, carrying my semen in her blouse.

"Are you sure?" Constance asked.

"Absolutely. Beyond the fact that I will not ask you to be my personal cum courier," I said, "I think I want to do it in the lab where we don't have to be in control of any variables. It's worth some discomfort of my surroundings to get it done right. We have enough to worry about. We don't need to worry whether or not we're keeping my sample at room temperature."

"Well, how long do you think it will take you?" she asked. "Dr. Leya said the earlier the better, since it has to sit at room temperature for a while before she can shoot it up in me."

Uninitiated to the insemination club, I had previously believed artificial or intrauterine insemination would be a less cliché version of the sperm in a turkey baster myth. Toxic shock stands between that dream and the reality, however, which has a technician spin the liquefied sperm down to a concentrated, elite swim team of the most viable athletes to bring home the baby-making gold. After being diluted with a bit of pink saline, they are finally ready for use.

I had no idea how long producing the sample would take. Would there be more screaming children on the cusp of vaccination to contend with? Would the hospital bathroom smell like a freshly mopped floor or more reminiscent of a stale, death-ridden nursing home? Would I once again be able to find that special place, that area of the brain accessed only when in severe pain, where I hid the first two times?

"Will getting there at six-thirty be early enough?" Constance asked, grabbing my arm before escorting me out of the elevator.

"That's when the lab opens," I said. "I guess I'll just have to make good use of my time."

When Dr. Leya inserted the thirteen-inch catheter containing the diluted pink mixture that once was my semen, now our great baby hope, into Constance's uterus, her eyes bulged and an audible gasp fled from her lips. I grabbed her hand and squeezed, collapsing my mammoth palm around her apple-size fist, and tried to sustain eye contact with my wife at the possible moment of conception. Her eyes were sealed, only unlike a normal climax and the other thousands of possible conception moments we had shared in seven years, they were not sealed as a result of pleasure.

"It's like when a man gets kicked in the groin," Dr. Leya said. "That's exactly what you're feeling right now. Like you just got kicked in the testicles. I know it hurts."

Before the insemination Dr. Leya removed the catheter

from its sleeve and showed me the vial with my name written on it. "Matthew Miller," she said with a smile. "That's
you, yes?"

"Yep, that's the guy," I said. "That's our baby daddy."

Dr. Leya pulled the stirrups from the exam table and positioned Constance's feet in them while she divulged that sometimes insemination is a 1-2-3 process that is quite easy for all
involved depending on how accessible the uterus is at any
given moment.

"Otherwise it's a 4-5-6 process and I'll have to use a dila-
tor," she said. Thankfully, it was the former, and with one swift
kick to the testicles, the deed was done. "Wow, Constance.
That was good for you and it was good for me," Dr. Leya said.

Earlier that morning I walked out of the hospital bathroom clutching a hazardous materials bag housing my sample.
Marked by a series of four partial red circles, devil horns
reconfigured into the shape of a daisy, my bag of sin was the
lone physical scar incurred during my escape from hell. Chin
dragging and eyes averting any and every gaze, I first spotted
the uniform white shoes of a nurse before I looked up to confirm her bleach blond existence.

"I'll take that for you," she said, snatching the bag from my
hand and placing my potential on an unsteady ledge.

"Thanks," I said, expressing my gratitude.

By the time we made it up to Dr. Leya's office on the third
floor and settled into the waiting room chairs, I couldn't escape

my masturbatory hell via the Cormac McCarthy novel I was reading. Life was bleak and strange, but Cormac McCarthy's world, illuminated by the fluorescent lights pissing down on us from the drop ceiling, was a bale of straw strapped to the back of a camel with a herniated disc.

We had at least an hour before the wash and spin cycles were completed on my sample, before the semen laundry was finished, and we needed to escape the artificial sperm-meets-egg setting for an edible egg reprieve.

We drove through Evanston's commuter traffic, stopping and starting and inching toward Le Peep for breakfast as construction workers blasted air into huge holes in the sidewalk. Dirt flew up into the sky, scattering on the uneven chunks of asphalt. Frost had blanketed the ground six nights in a row, and in the dirt I took solace, knowing this obliterated topsoil would not regain its fertile status for another six months.

"How did you do it?" Constance asked.

"I don't know. I huddled on the floor. I sat on my jeans. I tried not to think about anything. I was a machine, and I felt like a machine."

"Did you really have to concentrate or did you go to a special place?"

"Both," I said. "I was really concentrating inside my special place. I feel weird and gross. I feel the way you feel the day after a funeral. When you've cried a lot before going to bed. Like every person here eating their eggs and laughing around us has no idea what we're going through, and all I want is absolute silence. I wish I could lock myself in the movie theater all day and have nobody speak to me."

Post insemination we had to wait fifteen minutes for the injection to settle. I held Constance's hand and we talked about how easy it would be to mix up samples, especially with a last name as innocuous as "Miller."

"How are your testicles feeling?" I asked.

"Okay," Constance replied with a slight wince. "It's a different feeling than any other kind of nausea I've ever had. It feels like genitalia nausea. Like my genitals need to throw up."

"Genausea," I said. "It will go away, but not for a while. It feels like your whole body got turned inside out. It's so funny that you've always asked me what it felt like to be kicked in the nuts and now you know. I'm just so happy for you."

"If we were on *All My Children*, getting inseminated in Pine Valley Hospital, one of our exes would have snuck into the lab and swapped the samples," Constance said. Then, with a knock on the door, Dr. Leya released us. I watched Constance put herself back together again, pulling up her tights and skirt, pushing each arm through her knee-length black coat. Anyone looking at us as we left the hospital might have assumed we were young professionals, perhaps even doctors, leaving for an important appointment instead of leaving from one.

Our postnoncoital bliss was rapid, and within 10 minutes Constance dropped me off at work. I craved my dark movie theater of silence or a pillow over my head, but instead I repeatedly left my desk to stand in the hidden bathroom tucked in the conference room. I just stood there, unmoved, not tempted to unravel the peeling paint on the pipes or to give myself a glance in the mirror. I was unraveling, and I needed a room of my own. That day, the last day of November—insemination day—my room had a toilet and, courtesy of an unfortunate bottle of spray deodorizer, an odor reminiscent of poop in a peach patch.

Chapter 21

· ·

Tourists, Birthdays, and the Red Blood of Failure

Mom and Dad sat on the sofa with the puppies strewn across their laps like unconscious toddlers. A Christmas movie starring Matthew Broderick was on television, and it was reaching a noisy climax as we waited for Constance to finish getting ready. Despite the snowstorm, we were committed to our scenic trip down Lakeshore Drive to give my mom a good look at Chicago at Christmas en route to Shedd Aquarium. This was only the third time my parents had visited us in Chicago, and I wanted to make sure they understood why I was here—why Chicago was a better fit for my life.

Perhaps it was the unearthly way Matthew Broderick's neck appeared to bloom directly out of his chest cavity. Perhaps it was his creepy, lecherous guidance counselor meets Papa Smurf performance. Either way, turning away from the intoxicatingly insipid film when Constance called for me flipped my annoyance switch. What could possibly be more important than this? Who would win the speed-skating competition between Broderick and Danny DeVito? Would Christmas in this annoying suburb be ruined?

As it turned out, it would be. And there are worse things than missing a rare opportunity to see Danny DeVito speed skating.

Confidence or ignorance fueled me as I opened the door to the bathroom, expecting to quickly grab a roll of just-out-of-reach toilet paper for my short-armed wife and return in time for the skating. Instead of the comical scenario I expected—one in which Constance was dangling off the toilet, hair falling over her face like tinsel and trying to reach the paper cabinet on her own—I saw a red-soaked wad of white cotton being held aloft like a gruesome exhibit on some tacky cop show.

"It didn't work," she said. "I got my period. The insemination didn't work."

"Yeah, I see that," I said as I dipped to my knees in front of Constance. Wrapping my arms around her, she began to cry, and I began to tuck my anger deeper inside my body, past my stomach and into my toes. One of us had to remain strong because I didn't want our unified weakness to take us to that place where sympathy ends and fighting begins. As a way to make sense of the world, I preferred to place blame the way some people place phone calls, and that blame once again was piled onto my shoulders.

I wanted the one who was bleeding, to be the one feeling untainted love on our bathroom floor even if the urge to vomit and scream were foremost inside of me. "It's okay, baby," I said. "You know, it was just the first time. We'll get there."

"I know," she said. "But this just means we have to do it all over again. You have to jerk off into a cup again, maybe twice, and I have to get another ultrasound. And I don't want to do injectibles and if the next one doesn't work I have to take a shot in the butt every single day."

"I'm so sorry," I said. "It really sucks, and I'm so tired of waiting for this, but all it means is that I get another month of just me and you, and I don't think that's so bad at all." Jeans gathered at her ankles, Constance leaned tighter into my squeeze to the point where I could no longer tell where my black hooded sweatshirt ended and her turtleneck sweater began. Cheek to cheek, I nudged her head playfully and then lifted her chin into my hand. We kissed on the toilet, hovering over the remains of something that was nothing but something that meant everything.

"If I have to give you a shot every day, I promise to make it fun," I said. "Like, I'll pretend that you're terribly diabetic and the daily shots of insulin I administer will be the thin line that separates you from death."

Tears dropped from Constance's eyes more rapidly as she began to smile. "I'd really like that," she said.

Five minutes had passed since I left the living room, and my parents probably thought we had taken to having a rude quickie before our trip to the museum. Any other time they could have been right, but not today, and I had to let them know. Somehow we had to find the faces that shielded our disappointment and allowed us to function in public places brimming with screaming children that would never be ours. My birthday was three days away, twenty-nine was nigh, and that was the day Dr. Leya earmarked for pregnancy test, if there was no blood. But there was blood.

There will be blood, I thought, *there will always be blood.*

My chances to be a dad before the age of thirty was now limited to successes in one of the next three months.

Constance and I broke our embrace, and she flushed the toilet as I walked down the hallway to the living room. Credits rolled up the television screen as a Christmas carol blared without much joy. It was over and I missed it already.

"Dad, I bought bologna and plain potato chips for you if you want them for lunch," I said. "Mom, Constance just got her period."

∽——∾

"When do you want to do the test, Matty?" Constance asked as she plucked her eyebrows with her free hand, the gray cell phone wedged between her ear and shoulder. With my head propped on the smooth, frigid foot of our steel bed, I watched her in the bathroom but said nothing. She would have looked at home behind the wheel of an SUV driving a carload of suburban tots to private school. Moping face engaged; I would have looked at home in a Tennessee Williams revival.

Dr. Leya needed an exact date in order to replace the lab instructions for my semen analysis that Hazel the dog had eaten yesterday morning. One ten-minute shower and two unattended dogs resulted in a pile of excrement and shreds of green prescription paper strewn across the hardwood floors. The only legible, and apparently inedible, word left was *semen*. Since I had no choice but to remove the foulness in her absence, calling the doctor to tell her the dog ate my lab work fell upon Constance's shoulders.

A clinical study of my semen was needed again, for a third time, to give Dr. Leya her first personal look at my goods to get a clearer picture of why we remained not pregnant. Also, my first urologist didn't test the morphology from either sample I generated. For all we knew my sperm could have had mutant heads shaped like milk-dunked Keebler elves. Testing the morphology would give Dr. Leya a better idea if my sperm had the shape necessary to penetrate Constance's eggs. Testing the morphology would give me another chance to masturbate in public; the perfect method to taint my pre-Christmas vacation—once filled with cocoa, Lifetime movies, and biscotti—with some good old-fashioned trauma.

I closed my eyes and immediately fell back into a light

sleep. I began to dream I was standing in a grove of red delicious apple trees with wiggly sperm dangling from the limbs in lieu of fruit. I gripped a basket in one hand, and with my other hand, which was now a giant lobster claw, I picked them off one by one, placing loads of sperm into my plastic-lined basket.

"It's his birthday on Tuesday," I heard Constance say to Dr. Leya as she walked into the bedroom and startled me from my brief slumber. "Yeah, I know, right? What timing." Constance walked back into the bathroom and immediately began plucking errant hairs above her left eye to streamline her thick Italian growth. "Yeah, I guess that could work. That would be three days after his birthday. Hey, Matty, how about Friday?"

"Whatever," I said. "Friday is fine."

Friday wasn't fine. Friday was perhaps the worst day I could foresee in which to do my sample at the lab, but I couldn't determine a better day in the near or distant future, so Friday it would remain.

Semen analyses, it seemed, had no good days in which to be done. Six times in ten months, two at home, four at the lab. Produce a sample, aim into cup, expect bad news.

"God, I don't want to do this," I said. "Not at Christmastime."

"Will anything make it easier?" Constance asked.

"I know I said I'd never do this to you, but can you carry my semen to the lab in your bra? I just can't do it in the bathroom again. I can't take another person knocking on the door or trying to escape the cacophony of crying babies while I'm doing my thing. I just can't and please don't make me."

"You got it," she said. "I'm so sorry you have to do this again, especially on the week of your birthday, but I promise I'll make it fun. You know, since we'll be home and all."

Constance winked at me and sent a shiver throughout my body. She would be the John Stockton to my Karl Malone, the sexy Edge to my reluctant Bono, and her assist would spell the difference between postmasturbatory bathroom tears and unexpected pleasure.

She was beautiful music to my ears.

Chapter 22

· ·

Cocktails, IUI #2, and the Flat Tire That Obviously Hated Infertile People

"*Here's a couple of* anecdotes for your writing," Dr. Leya said. "I won't tell you names or anything, but there was one time a guy elected to produce his sample in my office, and right during the middle of it, the window washers came right down the side of the building and stopped in front of the window. Luckily he was so good-natured about it, but I mean, what are the chances? They wash the windows here twice a year!"

On another occasion, when Dr. Leya told another in-office masturbator that she had some *Playboy* magazines in the event he needed them to produce his sample, the man's wife said, "He won't need a magazine, just a mirror. Watching himself is all he really needs to get off."

Until that morning, Dr. Leya thought I was a professional musician because I once told her my band was playing at the Illinois State Fair. Had I known I had misled her to believe a dream I always wished was real, I would have taken more care to show up at appointments in skinny jeans and dirty T-shirts smelling like pot smoke and caked-on sweat. Dressed in a collared white and black shirt with a smooth black shirt over the top, however, brought an embarrassingly coy smile to her face.

"Oh, my gosh, you look so sharp," she said. "Did you trim your beard or get new glasses or something? Man, you look sharp."

It was a bit uncomfortable to see Dr. Leya's enthusiasm for my appearance, but I informed her that the only change in me was that I actually got dressed for that morning's appointment.

"Usually I get dressed afterward, but I'm going straight to work from here," I said, at which point she inquired about my job, and I told her about the newspaper syndicate for which I worked, as well as my blog about our infertility adventures, and the recent book deal I had signed.

"That's so great," she said, repeatedly fishing her ultrasound wand around Constance's vagina in search of our eggs. "One of the ovaries is always harder to find, but it looks like you've got two good eggs this month, maybe three. That third one, there on the left side, might be a little small to be ovulated."

Constance's face filled with discomfort as Dr. Leya pushed the wand back to the left side to measure the size of the third egg. "It's sixteen, it might work. And you know, now that I think about it, there really are no books or anything like that for men going through this," Dr. Leya said, removing the ultrasound wand from inside my wife. "That's going to be a huge help for so many people."

Dr. Leya removed the condom covering the end of the wand and dropped it into the hazardous materials bin along with her rubber gloves. "Okay, so we'll do the insem tomorrow morning, sound good?"

Constance and I had made the decision to wait until our new insurance took effect in January to go ahead with more procedures that were not covered under our current plan. Saving five hundred dollars seemed tantamount to one more month of insemination, which by now we had little faith in as our silver bullet.

Straight-up sex with Clomid for one more month, and then we'd move on to monthly inseminations and injectibles, and all of it would be on the tab of our new insurance company.

But when Dr. Leya posed the question, Constance cast her doe eyes in my direction and I, equally caught off guard, cast my own doelike glance back at her. When the glances collided, they exploded into a gnarly blinding light that erased all previous discussions on the matter and brought us back to the beginning. It was as if Dr. Leya had accidentally revealed herself as an alien reproductive endocrinologist and Will Smith and Tommy Lee Jones had shown up to wipe our minds clear all of that had come before.

"It's up to you, Matty," Constance said. Another day masturbating into a cup at the lab. Another day locked inside my cocoon of public self-pleasure hell. Answers are easy when you're selfish, but as much as the onus fell on me to produce another manual sample, it solely wasn't about my needs for a comfortable emission. Every time we skipped a step or missed a possible chance I didn't think about the money we saved; I thought about the baby we gave up.

"Actually, I think it's up to us," I said.

Dr. Leya clutched her chest as if her heart had been pierced by the bow of cupid himself and she would, at any moment, collapse in pool of her own blood. "Oh, you guys, I love that," she said. "That's so sweet. It's so nice to see you both in this together. Constance, get dressed and you guys can talk it over and then just meet me in my office."

Before she exited, I began to unfold Constance's underwear and pantyhose that were piled on my lap. After she opened the door, Dr. Leya turned back and said, "You know, you can just do it the old-fashioned way if you want for this month. It's up to you guys," she said, her last words clipped by the soft suck of the closing door.

"What do you think?" Constance asked as she folded up the paper blanket that had shielded her private parts from clear view.

"I think we should just go ahead and do it," I said. "I mean, we haven't even been billed for the first insemination at this point, so we'll have plenty of time to save up for it."

"Are you okay with splooging into a cup again tomorrow?" she asked.

"Yes, but we're doing it at home."

"Deal," she said. Constance dipped her toes into her pantyhose and began encasing her legs with them, emitting audible "uh" noises that sounded like the grunts of a belligerent child. I began to playfully mimic her as she shifted left to right, rolling them up her thighs.

"Are you making fun of me?"

"Yes," I said. "I think it's so funny you put your pantyhose on before we leave the house only to take them off ten minutes later."

"It's more comfortable," Constance said, pulling them up over her stomach and finally pulling down her skirt. "Plus they're easier to put on the second time." I continued to replicate her grunts as we put on our winter coats, gloves, and scarves. "I love you, Matty."

"I love you, Constance," I said, before throwing in two more mocking "uhs" for good measure as we walked out the door.

⌐‿⌐

"What time is it?" I queried, as Constance mined for the alarm clock beneath a pile of pillows and puppies.

"It's six-thirty!" she said.

"What?" I shouted. "What the hell, Constance? We have to be at the lab by seven."

"I know, I'm sorry. I thought it was earlier. I was just tired."

Like a martyr on speed, I jumped out of bed and ran to the bathroom across the hall. The swifter I got out of bed and got a move on, the more it would underscore my superior annoyance in regard to Constance's alarm clock follies.

Unsure what to do first, get dressed or masturbate, I opted to brush my teeth, to allow the electric buzz to enter my mouth and shake me awake before I revised our game plan. Constance fed the dogs and took them out for their morning bathroom time while I leapt into action. We would not make it to the lab by seven, that was a certainty, but if we both did the minimum to look presentable, I could make it happen pretty quickly when necessary and we could definitely be there by seven-twenty barring an unusual traffic flow.

"Matty?" Constance yelled over the top of our security system's three consecutive beeps, followed by a monotone voice intoning, "Front door." It was an unnecessary reminder that indeed, Constance just came back into the building. Shutting off the automated messages of the alarm would require reading the instruction manual or calling our security company, and neither seemed any less annoying of a proposition than living with constant verbal reminders of which door we were entering or exiting.

"What's wrong now?" I asked.

"We have a flat tire."

"Again?" I whined. It had been only a month since we re-placed two tires on our car following an unfixable flat, and now, with a sample to produce and deadline to meet, our car, much like our spirits, once again had deflated. "Well, I defi-nitely can't do the sample until the tire is fixed because I don't know how long it will take. We can't leave the semen out for too long."

Clad only in boxer shorts, I put on my coat, hat and gloves. Bending at the waist to pull my slip-on shoes onto my cold, large feet, I realized pants would be not only appropriate, but also necessary. I grabbed my favorite Princeton jogging pants, put them on, and opened the front door.

"Front door," the security system chimed again, louder and more aggressive sounding now that I was standing two feet from the auditory base, with little to no patience in reserve.

"Nothing like changing a flat tire in the freezing cold to set the masturbatory mood," I said, slamming the thick black door behind me, which sent an audible shiver through the hallway.

Twenty minutes later, I still couldn't get the lug nuts to budge. Push-up fueled muscles were no match for the air-powered wrenches at the tire center. After the last flat, they rotated all of the tires and strapped our wheels to the car as if any level of tightness below irremovable would put our PT Cruiser in grave danger of wheels flying off midtraffic.

"I can't believe they put them on so tight," Constance said. "What the heck are older people supposed to do? Or even me? I couldn't do it at all."

"They aren't even loosening," I yelled as I gave the tire iron one swift kick, which caused it to swing around and collide with my left femur. "Ouch," I yelled. "I hate this damn car! I hate cars. I hate this. I hate the snow, and I hate jerking off into a cup."

Every minute the tire remained fastened to the wheelbase put us in danger of blowing our chance at receiving our insemination this month. Constance called Dr. Leya to let her know our situation, and she said we had to be at the lab no later than eight because she had an unmovable appointment at ten AM downtown.

"You know, Matty," Constance said as she dug her fingers into my stiff shoulders, "I hate saying stuff like this because I don't believe in fate, but maybe it's just not meant to be this month."

Fate didn't exist for us, and I didn't exist for it. Eighteen consecutive months of not meant to be only strengthened my belief that nothing is meant to be and everything is chance. Sweat beads on my forehead froze into white chalk. A roofing crew down the street unloaded a load of gray shingles wrapped in white plastic, tossing oversized bundles over their shoulders and dropping them on the front lawn of our neighbor's house.

My dad would have fixed this flat in a blink, I thought.

Maybe the only thing that isn't meant to be is my being a father.

"You could always ask one of those roofers to help you get the lug nuts loose," Constance said. "I'm sure they'd help."

Never before had I felt this particular burn—my shoulders, my back, my forearms, my butt—but with Constance's words, that intense burn turned internal. Maybe it was an unavoidable deep-seated hypermasculinity. Maybe it was years of exposure to my father's stubborn pride, being a sidekick on his quest to keep the legend of his own hypermasculinity intact.

For in Chicagoland, they say, on his knees in the snow and grime, Matt Miller's muscles, like the Grinch's heart upon seeing the happy Whos on Christmas, grew three sizes that day. And the minute his muscles didn't feel quite so tight, he would unleash his load before dawn's morning light.

"Matty, you did it!" Constance shrieked as the first lug nut began its backward descent. Counterclockwise, each one fell to my newfound power, and eight minutes later I placed the mini spare donut where the full-size flat had been, and lowered the car back to the ground.

"Let's do this," I said, tossing the tire iron into the trunk and slamming the lid. Control of my seminal destiny and my reproductive future had no ties to flats, fates, or fitness. I controlled my own future, and my future had a date with a factory-sealed plastic cup that stood waiting on our bedside table.

She dipped her hand into her bra and pulled out the plastic cup that housed my semen. "Keep it warm in your hands," Constance said. "Take off your glove and hold it tight. You don't want to expose it to the elements."

Snow began to fall as we pulled into the circle drive; a thin sheet of powder already covered the walkway leading to the lab. I took off my right lamb's wool glove, stuck it in the side of the passenger door, and grabbed my sample from her hand.

"You know, maybe it's good luck," Constance said. "I was born in a terrible snowstorm. Maybe this is a good thing." I, too, was born in a snowstorm, but I didn't tell her that. I didn't want to jinx any amount of goodwill being offered by the cosmos on this otherwise appalling day.

Outside the lab stood a giant cardboard cutout of the Academy Awards statue outfitted in matte gold paint. White paper, outlining the lab's holiday hours, was taped to the spot where the statue's hands would have been had the cutout been anatomically correct. In the heat of the stressful morning, the inanity of the sign, which had no correlation to phlebotomy or urine collection, pushed me beyond my limit for nonsense. I kicked the feet of the statue on my way into the lab, and the Oscar wavered like a Weeble, wobbling but never falling down.

Resurrection Hospital's lab offered entrants a number, as if visitors were returning defective merchandise to a major retail outlet. Fitting, since I was indeed delivering defective merchandise to be spun into something better than I could have created on my own. I removed my outerwear, save for my fitted cap, and set the semen sample on a table next to my chair. I wrapped my lab order around the cup to shield others from its controversial contents. Time: eight-ten AM. Three people remained ahead of me in the wait to register. Unfamiliar with the needs of semen outside the body, I wasn't sure how long it could sit there and still be a viable sample. So, when the only woman registering patients halted her work and dialed her pregnant friend on the phone to hold a noisy catch-up session, I grabbed my semen and walked up to the counter. She made no eye contact with me, nothing to acknowledge my presence, so I produced a fake annoying cough to announce, passive-aggressively, that I had needs that superseded her personal expression.

"Hi, I have a time-sensitive sample here, and I was . . ."

"Sir, take a number and I'll be with you," she said, keeping her eyes fixed on the desktop to avoid my sullen glare. Numbered waiting routines were familiar to me, and I didn't take kindly to her condescending tone or her refusal to cease a personal phone call to answer my question.

"I have a number, but I also have to get this to my doctor right away," I said. Raising my semen to her eye level, I swirled it around the cup to show her that my sample was ready to become baby-making material.

"Sir, they just say it's time sensitive. I'll be with you in a few minutes." I returned to my seat and listened to her wrap up her conversation. Eight minutes later, my sample was in a plastic bag with my name on it.

"Just initial here and here," she said, "to give clearance to your sample, and then call your doctor in about an hour. It'll be ready then."

Constance and I put back on our winter gear and headed out the door.

"God, I hate that statue," I said.

"Do you want to get some breakfast?" she asked. "Before they shoot you up inside of me."

"Yeah, let's get out of here. I need some Jamba Juice."

Powdery film from the wheat grass shot clung to my tongue and a bit of pulp from the orange-wedge chaser was stuck between my crooked front teeth. Constance winced as the catheter inserted the good sperm past her cervix. I pushed my tongue between the crevice in my teeth, trying to force free the fruity remnant. Our eyes met when my face contorted into a lopsided snarl, and I immediately canceled my effort and forced a shy smile. Conception could not have occurred at that exact moment, but it was the only moment we would get. And my intention was to stare into my wife's eyes. Artificial, manual, bed, or exam table, I no longer cared how the baby was made, but I did long to have a connection of sorts at the time it happened.

"All right," Dr. Leya said. "You'll just need to lie there with your feet on the platform for fifteen minutes. But I actually got the results of your analysis back, so let me grab those and I'll be right back."

Pessimism runs through my family like big feet and a penchant for Doritos, and I had been to enough doctors to know the forthcoming news would be bad. Had the news been cheery, Dr. Leya would have announced it before discussing the results with me in the room where my sperm currently were making their impossible journey. Perhaps she wanted to give them a head start before bashing them for their nonconformity.

"Well, the morphology is great. Thirty-five percent, and anything above fifteen percent is fine. Your motility is fine, too, as is the volume and the number of sperm swimming in the right direction. The problem is the count. This time, it was only two million, and we're looking for a count between twenty and eighty million to conceive."

"That's so odd," Constance said. "Last time you had it done it was sixty million, and that was only ten months ago, right?"

"Yeah," I said. "Everything was fine then." A war raged inside my body, and it was something I feared from the start. Constance said time and again that we weren't looking for a place to lay blame, but in my mind I had been covering myself in glue for the last eighteen months, knowing that eventually blame for our infertility would stick to my shoulders, back, legs, and genitals. Blame was my addiction and instilled in me a sense of right and wrong. I wanted to be wrong, because I was tired of everything being scientifically right when everything was decidedly not right.

Troops of sperm, sent out to battle month after month, were losing the battle of the bulge to a greater, unknown force inside me. Finally, I had a target at which to aim the self-inflicted drive-by shootings constantly firing in my head.

"Well, counts are pretty unpredictable," Dr. Leya said. "But that's a big drop-off, which could signal a problem. It could be a varicocele, which is pretty common, and a urologist could treat that."

"How could it have changed so much so quickly?" I asked.

"Well, sperm quality goes back to about the previous four months," she said. "What you were doing four months ago can affect the count today, and it takes about that long to correct, too. Did you have any major changes?"

Twelve, eight, four months: life had been an embedded canker sore for the past year, annoying yet tolerable, and I knew the only things that had truly changed had changed in my mind.

"Not really," I said. "I mean, a little more stress, but my diet is the same, my exercise habits are the same. I can't think of anything catastrophic."

"Sometimes it just happens. So, here's the card for a urologist in this building. If the period doesn't come this month, then you don't have to worry about it. But if it does, I want you to go in for these blood tests to check your testosterone, FSH (follicle stimulating hormone)—everything that could be lowering your count."

FSH, she said, is essentially estrogen, and too much of it in a man can spark the onset of the male equivalent of menopause.

I could be turning sterile ejaculation by ejaculation.

Emasculated in an instant, punched in the groin by its anti-reproductive behavior, I turned my eyes away from Dr. Leya and Constance and focused on the diagram of a cancer-ridden vagina sitting next to the sink. Tumors filled the illustrated fallopian tubes like tiny bulbous brains. My mother-in-law's rectum and colon were filled with these thoughtless lumps, and as I stood there, unresponsive to the news I had just received, I said a little prayer to myself.

Please, whoever is listening, make Susan's butt cancer go away and make sure I'm not turning sterile at twenty-nine.

I should have engaged in a fit of laughter at my own expense as I prayed to an illustrated vagina, but I didn't laugh because it wasn't funny. It felt disingenuous to pray in the presence of science, but I had no choice. I had not prayed, in a formal sense, since the first time Susan had cancer, and my desperation once again led me to remove myself from my brain and live on a prayer. Either I was becoming sterile or I wasn't. Either Susan was going to recover from her cancer or she wasn't. Shuffling my feet from side to side, I removed my eyes from the diseased vagina and looked at Constance.

"Do you have any questions?" Dr. Leya asked.

Question number one was "Should I stop masturbating?" Question number two was "Can it be fixed?" Question number three was "What went wrong?" None of them were asked, though, because as eager as I was to blame myself, to shoulder the responsibility and take charge of the remedy, I wasn't ready for definitive answers about the long-term. I still wanted to believe every condition was fixable, even if my sperm were en route to extinction. I still wanted to believe our childlessness could be fixed.

"No, I guess we'll just have to see what happens," I said. "But it does concern me that my count has fallen so far so quickly."

"Remember, it is very likely temporary," Dr. Leya said. "We'll figure it out. Just give it time."

Constance stayed on the exam table for ten more minutes while the two million sperm tried their best to do what sixty million could have done better. After Dr. Leya departed, she wanted to walk me through it, to force me to put into words and dissect what depleted sperm meant to me and for us.

"I don't want to talk about it right now," I said. "I just want to think." This wasn't like the flat tire, and there was no way to Grinch myself out of this predicament by making my sperm grow three sizes that day. I could not prove my worth by thinking my count higher just to save masculine face. What it meant to me was I had once again failed my body somehow. Maybe it was my former obesity, maybe it was my current antiobesity; either way, I knew I had failed. And even though we were unsuccessful in getting pregnant back when the count was elevated, it felt like the inseminations in conjunction with the Clomid would have been a sure shot if not for me.

We left the hospital, and Constance drove me to the office through the increasingly slushy snow. It was the last day before New Year's break, a four-day vacation, and I knew that if I could get through this day, I would get a brand-new year and a brand-new start on the flipside.

Later that night at Whole Foods, we bombarded the shopping cart with pumpkin seeds, lentils, broccoli, tomatoes, quinoa, almonds, tilapia, decaf French roast, bee pollen, and Siberian ginseng.

"I need to find some carnitine, too," I said. "Although I can't for the life of me figure out if the carnitine will be in the supplement aisle or with the bulk herbs."

Before Constance picked me up from work, I did a quick Internet search for "sperm diet," which offered pages and pages of women and men in provocative poses but none dealing with the variety of sperm assistance I had in mind upon conjuring such a poorly worded phrase.

Work perks of the setting sort were few and far between in my constantly freezing, slightly dingy office space. Luxury of luxuries, however, my laptop was the only one in the company that faced a wall with no one behind me, so I was able to sneak a few lingering peeks before revising my search to "increase sperm count diet." Sifting through page after page created by the likes of fertility doctors, urologists, men with low sperm counts, and bored, tech-savvy hippies, I jotted down a quick list of every ingredient, vitamin, and practice known to help boost a weak sperm brigade.

I closed that search window and entered "varicousey" in a new tab. "Do you mean varicocele?" the automated return politely prompted, offering the benefit of the doubt that what I meant was actually something I knew.

It wasn't. Varicose veins in my testicles, like the purple rivers running down the legs of older women and emptying into an unattractive wasteland. Visions of spidery, wrinkled octogenarians in knee-length nightgowns flooded my head, and my testicles began to retreat into my body.

Varicocele: an abnormal enlargement of the veins around the scrotum, which decreases blood flow and, ultimately, sperm count. Roughly forty percent of infertile men have one. Until today, every bit of evidence, at least evidence of the official scientific variety, pointed to my sperm count hovering above the dead-center mark of normal. But that was prior to our second insemination, a morning that saw me wielding a tire iron, downing shots of wheat grass, and receiving a bit of juicy semen gossip that changed everything.

"How many pumpkin seeds do you think you'll need?"

Constance asked as she dipped the scoop into the bulk bin for the third time.

"I need to eat at least a quarter of a cup every day," I said.

"Do you even like pumpkin seeds?" she asked.

"I have no idea, but I guess it doesn't matter if I like them or not," I said as I scanned the bins for spelt and any other whole grain that looked slightly more edible than gravel. "Let's just hope my sperm have a hankering for them."

Three hours and one two hundred dollar expenditure later, I had all of the homeopathic makings to morph myself into the virile man I had always wanted to be. Money could not buy love or happiness, but I clung to the hope it could buy enough bee pollen to bring about a semen revival come 2008.

And perhaps, as a result, a baby before I turned thirty.

Chapter 23

· ·

Flashlights, Blood Streaks, and Text Messages from a Toilet

We had to use a flashlight to see for ourselves, but in the end both the darkness and the focused beam of light told the same cliché story. Insemination number two had failed us. Second verse, same as the first, and this once optimistic song was beginning to grate on my nerves. A sunny, uplifting Stevie Wonder composition reduced to something mocking and soulless, stripped of rhythm by a stiff-throated pop star.

Both the vanity lights and those encased in the small glass overhead fixture in the bathroom had been out for five days, and we couldn't find the source of their failure. We swapped out eco-friendly bulbs for standard incandescent bulbs I kept around in case a freak surge had caused all five to blow simultaneously. I checked circuit breakers to make sure they were in their correct and upright positions. Everything appeared to be on the up-and-up, but we chose not to call the condo developer and instead shower, shave, brush, and pee in complete darkness. Living without light was easier than dealing with unresponsive construction workers, and we both assumed the problem would either present itself or fix itself in due time.

"Matty, it's here!" Constance yelled from the bathroom. Yoga mats covered the small space between the kitchen island and the stove, and I was bent over tying my running shoes when she called. My bronchial infection–prone lungs made it impossible for me to run outdoors when the temperature dipped below forty-five degrees, and as a result, I had perfected a nearly flawless stride simulation in order to maintain my fitness indoors, sans treadmill. Our neighbors below didn't seem to mind as long as I limited my indoor runs to the kitchen, where the wood floors rarely creaked or moaned against my down steps cushioned by the yoga mat beneath my feet.

"Are you sure?" I asked as I walked into the dark bathroom. "I had such a vivid dream only two days ago that you were pregnant. It felt so real." Never before had I subconsciously conjured a scenario in which we had created a child, but two nights previous I had a dream of a stick, two lines, and uncontrollable sobbing. I woke up smiling and Constance woke up sad. Hormonal changes were occurring, but I couldn't help but feel optimistic in the face of her unexplainable grief. Unwilling to elevate more hopes than my own, I kept the prophetic dream and armchair diagnoses to myself. Instead, I hugged my wife and sang impromptu songs about her beautiful face until she began to feel better two days later.

"I'm pretty sure it's my period," Constance said, once again lifting a piece of toilet paper for me to inspect. "It's been light all day, but it definitely feels like there's a lot more coming right now."

"Let me look at it with the flashlight," I said. "I used it this morning and it worked great."

"What did you use it for this morning?" she asked while I pushed Cleo aside, a constant feline fixture on our bathroom countertop, and reached for the flashlight behind her wide, fluffy frame.

"I took a big poop and I wanted to see just how big it really was," I said, thankful for a shroud of darkness to hide my blushed cheeks.

"You are the strangest boy," Constance laughed, her boisterous chuckle a friendly firing squad taking aim at my self-conscious ego. Pop. Pop. Pop. "I can't believe you did that."

"What, I just wanted to know. It's impossible to monitor my bowel movements in this darkness." My thumb fumbled for the plastic hump that, when depressed, would shine a light on a wad of toilet paper marked with a map of our next steps. If there was blood, it meant more than no baby. It meant another trip to the urologist. It meant another intimidating, handsome stranger's hands on my balls and penis for further exploration as to why my sperm were on the brink of extinction. It meant more masturbating into plastic cups and more ultrasounds, shots, and pills for Constance. It meant more disappointed entries on my blog. It meant I was going to work on Monday instead of calling in sick to celebrate and to sleep for the first time with the knowledge and relief that the finish line of infertility finally had been crossed.

It meant no baby.

Slowly pressing the button on the flashlight, a weak ray of light shot out of the barrel and exploded in a burst of unmistakable red.

"Well, the flashlight doesn't lie," I said. "My poop was just as big as I thought it was, too." Constance laughed, I laughed, and her one flush of the toilet seemed to erase what had taken us days to surmount the month before. Babies weren't in our near future, and the only thing we could do at that point was to continue squinting and scanning, hoping that the fine print would indeed get us closer to fine.

"Who are you texting on the toilet?" I asked

"Krista," she said. "She was sure that my recent depression was because I was pregnant. She's been so sweet to me. I swear, she feels like she has as much riding on this as we do sometimes. We have the nicest friends. I don't know what we'd do without their support."

"I was so sure, too, just like Krista," I said. "I guess all lesbians think alike."

Later that day Constance solved the mystery of the dark bathroom. No power filled the vacuum, no deafening growl to alarm the dogs when she tried to clean up the mess left behind by the puppies' boredom-forced destruction of their own beds. Shortly thereafter she realized the puppies had turned off the circuit on the GFCI outlet outside the bathroom during one of the countless times Hazel body slammed Marcy into the wall—scuffs on the paint, a perfect DNA match for our out-of-control hounds' act of stupidity.

"Hey, Matty, the light works now. I fixed it."

"Oh, thank God," I said. "I'm tired of relying on the flashlight to be my eyes. I need a little more clarity than that." Perhaps the urologist would be ugly, and perhaps he would shower me with a little of the light I craved, but what I craved above all was clarity.

"My, how literary of you," Constance said. "Very profound."

"Oh, I was just talking about my poop." I said coyly. "I didn't want to have to use the flashlight again to get a good look. What were you talking about?"

Chapter 24

• •

Acupuncture, Afghanistan Babies, and the Urologist Who Wasn't George Clooney

Mary fumbled through her oversize purse, digging through a massive stack of postcards and makeup containers until she located the noisy plastic bag that was the target of her search. A yellow and orange printed scarf tucked into her stylish jean jacket accented a flawless, quirky look any actress worth her innovative salt would die for. Mary had grown up with calcium-deposit stained front teeth, plastic white glasses, and an artistic fashion sense that was her magnetic north, a clever method to draw attention away from the obvious foreshadowing that her adolescent awkwardness was simply a thin veneer for a soon-to-blossom, effortless beauty.

"Here you go, Matty," she said. "It's a late Christmas, but really-just-because gift. I'm sure you've seen this book. I think it's great. There's an inscription inside just for you guys."

Placing the bag down on a table in the far corner of Glenn's Diner, I clearly could see the familiar '50s-era illustration of a modern mother on the cover peeking out through the plastic bag. *Deceptively Delicious: Simple Secrets to Get Your Kids Eating Good Food* by Jessica Seinfeld.

Black Friday shopping had first led me to this book, when a particularly pushy woman amid scads of pushy women clamoring to get the latest video game for their kids pushed me face-first into a rack of discounted books. Fate it was not, but my innate fear of raising a fat kid bubbled to the surface, and combined with the irresistible illustrations of tomatoes and squash that adorned its pages, I inscribed the trendy tome upon the mental list of things to buy once we were pregnant.

> Dearest Matt & Constance:
>
> This book is:
>
> A vote of confidence that you will one day be cooking for 3+ . . .
>
> A belated Christmas gift.
>
> Given so that you can make the doughnuts on page 160 and have me over for snacks.
>
> Love always,
> Mary, 2008.

"Mary, that's so great," I said. "You are so thoughtful. I think that's remarkably sweet."

"I was so appreciative that you gave me the go-ahead yesterday, about the whole acupuncture thing. I just don't like to dawdle, but I really do think it could be good for you." The ponytailed waitress interrupted our discourse to fill the highball water glasses and remind her patrons that the chef was fresh out of scallops, a fact also inscribed in large, can't-miss block letters on the chalkboard lining the wall right above our table.

"You can always come to me with advice, Mar. You know that." In the nineteen months of our infertility, few people had shown modesty when offering advice. Mary had not been one of them, but she could no longer unnecessarily hold her tongue when she learned I was trying some out-of-the-box alternatives to cure my low sperm count. Her e-mail was passionate and, in typical Mary fashion, outlined three points of interest to justify her actions.

Dear Matty:

Okay, so I have refrained from saying absolutely *squat* about you and Constance's struggle with fertility. Why? Because:

1) Even though you write a candid blog about it, it's essentially none of my damned business.

2) You surely get *loads* of well-meaning but annoying advice already from friends, family, strangers, etc.

3) I don't really know what the fuck I'm talking about.

However.

I was just a few minutes ago working on an assignment that led me to www.fertilespirit.com. Before you click on it, lemme just say that I spent about 45 minutes reading the "success stories" tab. Matty, I'm telling you, just check it out.

When I was getting acupuncture last year on a regular basis, I flew into my doctor's office one day with a panic-stricken face. I had read an article about how acupuncture can lead directly to babies, since the body's qi becomes so unblocked, shiz starts flowing *real, real* freely. Everywhere. My doctor said that I was right to be worried, that yes, acupuncture is highly effective as a fertility treatment.

I assume you've checked this out, being the progressive couple you are. But you should read some of these stories at this website. Very similar accounts of people trying for many years with no luck and then they start seeing Dr. Ian and Bev and it's like, *POW*.

So there you have it. I've officially butted in and given totally unsolicited advice. But I just couldn't keep reading those testimonials and not let you know.

Love, Mar

"I'm actually going to spend some time at that site tonight," I said. "I've been considering acupuncture. My friend Holly gave me the card of someone who says she can 'cure' my infertility in three months' time, but I don't know." Aspects of acupuncture made sense to me, and I long suspected my body was out of whack due to the swing from obesity to normality. My hair fell out as a result of my extremes, and it made sense that my qi could be in need of realignment. But I wasn't totally sure I bought into the idea that qi existed, and I knew that even as I sat there saying I would look at the information, I knew that I probably wouldn't.

"How is everything going with you two?"

"You know, it just gets more bizarre every single day. This morning we went to have my blood tests done to figure out what happened to my sperm."

"Sixty million to only two million," Mary said. "That's not good, Matty."

"I know, but with all of the supplements and bee pollen and stuff, my, uh, output, really is different."

"I read about that on your blog," Mary said. "So how exactly is it different? Is it like spackle now? Or caulking?" Water dribbled out of my mouth and down the front of my button-down brown turtleneck sweater as I laughed so boisterously that the patrons across the room turned to make sure I wasn't in the midst of some brand of seizure.

It was true. Two Saturdays previous I noticed my semen had become a different entity since beginning my new regimen. Perhaps it was the frisky, unseasonably springlike air that filled our lungs as we walked the dogs to Starbucks as the sun rose for the first time in a week, the arrival of two sixty-degree days that unearthed our dormant debauchery. Perhaps it was the aphrodisiac properties of a gourmet chicken-and-leek soup Constance prepared for lunch while I wrote, punching keys on my silver laptop while she seductively sliced and rinsed the suggestive relatives of my favorite vegetable. Perhaps it was a random act of digestion-induced arousal as we cuddled next to each other on the sofa and watched a Rice Krispies Treats competition on the Food Network, one creation being an exact replica of downtown Baltimore filled with tall skyscrapers.

Regardless the reason, there simply wasn't enough time or the impetus to close the blinds. Afterward, as gravity did its work, I got my first good look at my goods post-sperm-count diet. "Look at it," I said, pointing at a body part somewhere below my belly button. "It's totally different."

"Whoa, it really is," Constance said, rolling onto her side with my T-shirt tucked between her legs. "It looks completely different."

Mary's analogy at lunch that day wasn't far off the mark. What was usually watery and translucent was now neither. It was drastically different from the many, many, many times I had seen it in the past, like looking into the mirror and suddenly having green eyes or a full head of curly brown hair.

"You and Constance must be getting mentally exhausted by this point," Mary said. "It seems like you'd about have to be. So much hope and letdown, and around and around."

"More than anything it's just an increasingly bizarre series of events that makes me question my own sanity," I said. "People tell me the strangest things. Like the phlebotomist this morning, when she asked why I was getting my blood drawn. I told her that we'd been trying to get pregnant for more than a year and a half with no luck. She then gave me a choice between my right and left arm. I said I didn't care. Then she asked me which hand I write with, and I told her my right and also thanked her for thinking of that because I'm a writer. Before I knew it, the other phlebotomist walked over and asked about my writing, my education, how far we were in our infertility treatment, and suddenly my life was open for discussion. They were little bombs careening out of the sky, and I was the ground below, moving farther along in the process than even we had. 'IVF is expensive and costs more than some houses,' they said, and I told them how lucky we were that our insurance covered it. Then the female phlebotomist told me about her son and daughter-in-law, whose cancer is in remission, but she's now infertile, and how they might hire a woman in Afghanistan to carry their child because it's only six thousand dollars compared to forty thousand in America."

"Excuse me?" Mary said. "Uh, what the hell was that about? Why would she tell you that story?"

"I have no idea, but it happens all the time. Most of the time it's people trying to help, but a lot of times, like this morning, it's utter nonsense and kind of upsetting. I had to keep myself from laughing as she poked and poked at my arm. I wasn't exactly sure what she was implying about our situation. Nothing probably. I had to stop myself from telling her that sometimes you get what you pay for and that it might be worth the extra to avoid having to go to Afghanistan multiple times just to reproduce."

Yeah, it's not like you can just ship your semen and eggs to Kabul," she said as the waitress approached our table to take our order. "Speaking of, I'm definitely getting an omelet for lunch."

With our insurance switch, moving from a PPO to an HMO, we had to abandon our current doctors at Swedish Covenant and designate a new primary care physician in order for us to continue seeing Dr. Leya and, ultimately, for me to make an appointment with the urologist to whom she referred me.

After Constance called and signed us up for a doctor who was a member of Dr. Leya's network, a critical step in receiving uninterrupted service, I called for an appointment with my new urologist, Dr. Sharp. After giving the woman on the phone every inch of my personal history, miles of digits and addresses and previous medical incidents, she informed me that the first available appointment was three weeks out.

Dr. Leya previously mentioned that she could do the exam herself, and has done so in the past, but had stopped offering the service because most men aren't comfortable with a woman doing the poking and prodding of their genitalia.

I was not most men, however, and I was not in a mood to wait around for a man to fondle my testicles when a woman could do the job just as easily. Perhaps it actually would be a preferable thing to drop my pants for Dr. Leya, I decided. She had become invested in us, and she knew what was going on, and I could save myself fifteen minutes of explanation and the dredging up of bad memories to satisfy a new doctor's interest. Telling the same story of a disappointing nineteen months had become tedious, and even though one shouldn't put all his eggs in one basket, we seemed to have more than enough eggs.

"Nah, I want you to see Sharp," Dr. Leya said. "He's the urology expert, and I really want to get a clear shot of what's happening down there. For now just head on down for your blood tests."

Dr. Sharp's office was in the east wing of the same hospital where Dr. Leya's office was located. I was armed with printouts of my blood tests, all of which came back showing normal levels of everything. I officially was not entering "manopause." My testosterone, progesterone, prolactin, FSH (follicle stimulating hormone), LH (luteinizing hormone), and pH levels were what every man should hope for but provided no insight into the drop of my count.

"What I was looking for was to see if you had gone into the male version of menopause," Dr. Leya said. "But all of your tests were great, which is a very good thing."

Now, it's been almost one year to the day after the first time I went to the urologist, when young handsome Dr. GQ, like a less annoying cast member of *Grey's Anatomy*, fondled my bits and instructed me, for the first time, to generate a sample in the hospital lab. The trauma of that day, huddled in the sterile, noisy hospital bathroom, seemed like it could not be surpassed or replicated, and that it was likely the worst of what was to come.

Thinking back on the wickedly naïve me from that day as I sat in the lobby of urologist number two made me feel old, like when seeing a group of high schoolers on the El train who suddenly look to be not a day older than twelve. Filling out the same informative forms, outlining my medical history, the health histories of my family, and the history of the last nineteen months, the whole process had somehow come full-circle, placing me right back where we were one year ago. As if I needed written affirmation that no progress had been made.

Butterflies on speed flew a heightened state of irritability in my stomach, a kamikaze fighter jet crashing into my upper half and toppling my gut and head.

Please let Dr. Sharp be old and ugly. I do not need another GQ *model inspecting my goods.*

Disrobing in front of strange medical men and showing a parade of doctors the scars of my obesity was a humiliation that conjured both the burn of tears and the urge to vomit on pristine white lab coats. The very least Dr. Sharp could contribute to my day was to agree to be unattractive. Ugly people, just by their mere presence, made me feel more secure about my own shortcomings.

"Do I know you from somewhere?" Dr. Sharp asked as he gripped my hand for the first time. I put my iPhone on top of my coat in the chair next to me to free my other hand, the screen still glowing with a *New York Times* story about the difficulty senators face on the road to the White House. His fingers were thin and short, his hands smooth and hairless, and I was grateful that my soon-to-be-painful prostate probe would be handled by such delicate small hands.

"I don't think so," I said, breathing deeply as I moved my gaze up to his face, the face of your everyday fifty-something man who would never be cast as lead doctor on a television drama. Relief came courtesy of his receding hairline, freckled face, and modest paunch.

He has no reason to judge me.

"You look so familiar, I swear I know you. You just look so artsy. Hard to forget a guy like you. Anyway, tell me what's up."

Our story unfolded again and again and again, in coffee shops, at wedding receptions, at the dentist's office, and there was no escape from talking about our infertility because we were almost thirty, married for over five years, and everyone wanted to know why we were so selfish as not to have kids as yet. It was defining who I had become in the present, and that new definition of me was no longer one I wanted clinging to my flesh.

"Do you have any STDs?"

"None."

"Multiple sexual partners?"

"No."

"Do you use marijuana? And be honest, because if you do that's a big one right there. Marijuana makes sperm lazy and stupid."

"No, I don't."

"Has your wife been receiving treatment?"

"Yes, from Dr. Leya."

"Joan is the best," he said, looking up from his chart, grinning like a child impressed by his mother's fame.

"We love her," I said. "She's been absolutely perfect. The best thing for a couple like us."

"Okay, then, drop your pants and shorts, and I'll give you a quick look and then a finger up the butt." His directness was refreshing, and it made sense that Dr. Leya and Dr. Sharp were intertwined, colleagues and friends who didn't administer wishful thinking or conjectures to vulnerable, desperate people willing to believe anything positive to be the gospel.

His fondling was brief and his intrusive finger under-lubricated, but in thirty seconds' time I was pulling my pants back up while Dr. Sharp began to scribble prescriptions.

"I need two semen analyses," he said, "one today if you've abstained for at least three days."

"I have," I said, nodding aggressively like the smartest kid in class, the kid who knew not to masturbate or have intercourse before going to the urologist. Knowledge that, like geometry, would not be applicable in real life. "I knew I'd have to do this."

"Okay, then, we'll get one today and one in seven weeks. Sperm is made seven weeks out, so we need to test where you are now and where you are then to see if you're on the rebound or holding steady." Blood tests, the same ones required by Dr. Leya, were to be performed again, as was a urine test. Out in the reception area, he handed me two cups and three prescriptions for lab tests.

"I saw you on as I walked in after rounds," he said, snapping his fingers in recognition of the light bulb that, after a lengthy darkness, had finally illuminated his memory of me. "You looked so artsy and tall and thin, I just knew you were my patient who Joan had described."

"Thanks! I'll definitely take that as a compliment," I said, shoving two semen cups into my coat pockets as I walked out the door toward the one-stall bathroom to the left of his office.

"Uh-uh. Sorry. Too late. No semen after noon. Sorry." Maria's round, scrunched face was in a permanent frown position from the moment I walked into the lab waiting room. First refusing to make eye contact with me while she watched CNN on the flat screen, she was now refusing to make eye contact with me out of fear, shoving the prescription back across the counter and dismissing me with a wave of her wrinkled hand.

"Excuse me?" I yelled. Producing the sample had been no easier than the first three hospital experiences, and I was in no mood to be sent home with a wasted cup of hard-fought semen.

"Right here. In paper, see? No semen after noon. Who told you to do this?"

"Dr. Sharp," I said, "upstairs in urology. I just produced the sample and brought it down."

"Nothing I can do. You have to come back tomorrow."

"Look, this isn't like a cup full of urine. I just can't go into the bathroom and make some more whenever I feel like it. I'd have to wait three days, come back, and do it again, and I refuse to do that. This is unacceptable."

"Let me call," she said, her eyes never yielding their fixation of inanimate objects that wouldn't yell or glare with the ferocity I was yelling and glaring. After a brief minute on the phone, in which she asked the lab if they still accept semen, a fact she knew to be false, she thanked them and hung up the phone.

"Sorry. Semen only between seven and noon."

"Unacceptable," I screamed, fighting the urge to grab the sample cup and throw it in her angry little face. Three other patients were in the waiting room, but I didn't care if they thought the semen guy had lost his mind. Nobody there knew what I had gone through to get to this point, and Maria didn't care to work with a fragile man to get his semen inspected for the fifth time. "I need to speak with a manager, and I will not leave until we get this figured out."

"Okay, sir," Maria said, picking up the phone and dialing the lab once again. "There's an angry man here with his semen sample and somebody told him to bring it in for testing this afternoon, but it's too late."

Silence.

"For infertility?" she asked me, allowing her eyes to greet mine for the first time.

"Yes, infertility," I said.

"Okay, that's good. I will tell him, and I will also call his doctor to tell him this is the last time we accept late semen. Okay, bye-bye."

"Here, fill out this form here to verify the facts about your sample and sign here and here."

"Thank you, Maria," I said, grabbing the pen from the table and scribbling the numeral "three" in the blank spot where it called for the number of days since my last ejaculation. Writing about my ejaculate, whether it was a full, complete, or partial, was a post-rage relief. Maria was not my friend, Maria did not care that my semen was now on its way to the microscope, but Maria had feared my postmasturbatory rage enough to do what I asked, and I was grateful. "I can't tell you how much this means to me. You get the gold star for today."

"Okay," she said. "That's fine. Just put the cup in the toxic bag here and then wait for your name to be called for your blood test. Your semen is done for today. Call your doctor on Monday for results."

Without pause, before I could gather my coat, the remaining prescription, and my insurance card, she dismissed my case.

"Number forty-three! Who's number forty-three? Forty-three? Okay. Forty-four?"

Chapter 25

· ·

Facebook, Braces, and a "Sopranos"-esque Ending

Orion stopped me on my way into the office, the faux fir-lined hood of my coat sandwiching my face like two ferrets. My one and a half mile walk to work through eight inches of snow burned cold through my boots, coat, sweater, and hat. "So, your cousin Jackie is pregnant, huh?" he said. Thawed by the frustration of another relative getting pregnant, my face went from cold to hot in the course of seven words.

"What?" I asked, pulling the earbuds from my canals. Radiohead was blasting art rock through my noise-canceling headphones, but even through the shredding guitars and high-pitched wailing, I heard his message loud and clear. I just didn't believe it.

"On Facebook, your cousin Jackie asked me to add her as a friend, and then yesterday she announced she was pregnant in the message area. You didn't know?"

"No," I said, "I didn't know. Eerie quietness, save for the hum of the industrial refrigerator and the El train passing behind our desks that always welcomed Orion and me into the office. That day my chilly indifference, as the tally of conceptions and births by first cousins during the time of our infertility rose to seven, made the stillness uncomfortable.

Dr. Leya instructed us to skip Clomid or inseminations for the month of January until I completed my visit with Dr. Sharp and we got a better look at why my count was so low or, optimistically, if it had risen from the barren levels. February was in jeopardy, too, if there wasn't any progress made as a result of my new sperm-boosting health routine.

"We don't really do IUI unless the count is at least five million," Dr. Leya said during our last visit, when I found out my sample during our second insemination had fallen below two million. Off the drugs and back to natural, Constance became imbalanced, and her hormone readjustments made her both cranky and sensitive.

Nobody in my family knew Jackie was pregnant before I told them, which wasn't a huge surprise. We knew very little about each other because we were relative strangers. Regardless of our feelings for one another, I couldn't imagine being afforded that same luxury, to do something so natural without every member of your family knowing your every failure. Few people could boast the familial support Constance and I did, and I couldn't be more grateful, but as the news bit

my frostbit skin that morning, I became sad for the first time
at the thought of being robbed of the unexpected moment, the
announcement of our surprise pregnancy, because everyone
knew we were trying and everybody knew that when we got
pregnant it would be a miracle.

Angie always knew how to save me, so I e-mailed her in
hopes that she could do it again on a day when I needed it as
much as I needed oxygen and Starbucks. When I was eight,
my eldest sister gave me the Heimlich maneuver when I
choked on a half-chewed vanilla wafer. When I was ten, she
took me driving with her blond stripper boyfriend, and I
crashed the car into a telephone pole going five miles per hour.
She gave me adventures and comfort, and while it wasn't her
job to talk me down off the ledge after our cousin achieved
something she deserved just as much as Constance and I did,
I needed her to save me.

And she did. Her words were those of someone who
understood, and I was so lucky that my greatest resource for
infertility patience was also my greatest cheerleader.

"I know what you mean about the waiting. It does suck and
it doesn't seem fair. I know in my heart that it will work out in
the end, so just keep your head up," said my sister. "Little Miss
Ali is living proof that it can happen, so don't give up yet. I
wish you didn't have to go through this, but it will only make
your relationship with the baby when it comes that much
more wonderful. I'm not saying I love Ali more than Chelsey,

but it is a different kind of love—the love of wanting something so bad and really appreciating it when it happens. I know at nineteen I didn't fully understand the miracle that Chelsey was to me. Having waited all these years for Ali, fifteen years, it becomes so much clearer. I know that you will have a beautiful baby coming your way soon. Maybe your wait is to help other people get through their rough times like you do in your blog and also with your book. You have inspired and helped a lot of people with this wait, and when the reward happens, it will be so much greater."

A handful of vitamins, the reimplementation of testicle icing, the Kombucha tea, the bee pollen, the daily orange, and the pumpkin seeds apparently were just what the Internet doctor ordered. Following three record-low months, two counts collected via inseminations and one via semen analysis, each resulting in a sperm count of 1.8 to 2 million, I got a call from Dr. Sharp that changed everything.

"Your tests aren't complete," he said, "we're still waiting on the morphology. But your count is twenty-three point eight million."

"Are you serious?" I asked, a surge of warmth marching into my blushing face. "I can't believe that."

"Yes, it's a great turnaround," he said. "Just keep doing what you're doing."

I had made a miraculous recovery. I was down for the count, sucker-punched below the belt by a dirty opponent, but a sperm-friendly diet and routine had picked my fellas off the floor and had me ready to go a few more rounds. I felt like a man again, like I had the virility to make a child possible.

Twenty-three million sperm, equivalent to the human population of Inner Mongolia, were present for my last analysis. I got the call at my desk, which was always awkward, since the trendy loft space where I wrote and edited offered few walls and no sound barriers to edit my personal time.

Once I found out I had achieved my mission it was so hard to be happy but not be able to tell everyone my great news. Its is the best news I'd had in a long time, on Valentine's Day to boot. Unlike the flowers sitting on my boss's desk, which signified her happiness for the day, there was no appropriate way for me to fly my flag of joy.

News like that was even tantamount to Constance's period still not arriving for the month. Light bleeding showed up to work on Monday afternoon and then decided to take Tuesday off for a much needed vaginal vacation.

"Do you think it was implantation bleeding?" I asked, hopeful that the small amount of blood that arrived was merely nature running its course.

"I have no idea," Constance said, fixing her hair in the bathroom mirror, adjusting her barrette to give more lift to the poof in the front of her head. "I don't feel pregnant, but we can take a test if you want."

To celebrate our period-free Valentine's Day, we chose to take the test once our romantic dinner of pad thai and chicken satay had been delivered. We placed plates around the table, a small glass of wine at the top of each setting, and Constance sat with the stick in her pocket.

"We're not going to look at it for five minutes," she said, popping open the Styrofoam hotdog container filled with steamed vegetable pot stickers. We finished all six, dipping them in a dark plum sauce and chewing in silence, and then Constance pulled out the test.

"Not even the hint of a second line," she said. I reached out for the test and held it up to the light, twisting it back and forth in the dimly lit living room in hopes that a faint mark would emerge at just the right angle.

"Nothing," I said, placing the test in the lid of the empty pot sticker box. "Wouldn't that have been a great ending?"

"Yeah," Constance said, grabbing my hand, squeezing the glazed wooden chopsticks into my palm. "It would have been the perfect ending."

❧

Dr. Washington's fingers yanked the wire strung through the lower brackets glued to my crooked teeth. Braces were my gift to myself, using the first half of my book advance, and after only one day of wearing them, a front bracket had popped loose, spinning and rattling against my teeth with the pronunciation of every word.

"Are you okay?" she asked, tugging the wire free and holding it up for me to see. "We'll get you fitted for rubber band brackets and a stronger wire today, too. You're making good progress."

Cheek separators were once again pushed between my lips, a thin plastic oval expanding my mouth beyond its opening limits. A plastic tongue depressor forced my tongue to the back of my throat to keep the enamel dry as the acid wash was applied and the bracket reglued. Being mildly claustrophobic, I had shoved Dr. Washington's assistant away from my face during the first application, pushing her gently into the utility tray that housed my brackets and wires, while the water pooled in the back of my throat and my heart rate elevated to a sprinter's beat.

"Charise, how was your Christmas?" Dr. Washington asked her assistant, who was holding the ultraviolet heat lamp while Dr. Washington forced my bracket into place.

"Girl, I got one of them Best Buy credit cards and got me a new flat screen. That's why I'm here working on a Saturday, 'cause I gotta pay that off now!"

"Charise, what were you thinking? You know if you can't pay for it, you just gotta walk out of the store."

"I couldn't do it. I knew I should have, but the kids wanted it so badly, and it was six months without interest. Now I've got five televisions in my house."

"Next time you're in that situation you call me and I'll tell you, 'Charise, walk away from the Best Buy.' I didn't go into any debt this Christmas. That's stupid. I got Denise what I could afford, and she was more than happy."

"I know, but you know how it is with kids. They always want something, and you always want to make them happy if you can."

"Do you have any kids?" Dr. Washington asked, smiling down on me from above, a sun above the clouds that would not part. My mouth was full of apparatuses and water, and my anxiety at having so much stuff and so many people in my face was causing my throat to constrict and my palms to sweat. After months of telling every person who asked about our infertility, after justifying our childlessness by espousing the details of our struggles to the point of weariness and opening our sores for everyone we knew to pick, I now was strapped in a massage chair, my head tilted back as cartoons played on the flat screen in front of my chair, without the option to speak. I didn't shrug or nod or shake to parlay any information about my life to a stranger who wouldn't understand anyway. She had a child, I didn't. She could speak, I couldn't. I didn't want to tell her anything about who I was or what we'd been through, and I didn't want to hear two more words about her daughter's favorite new stuffed dog. I just wanted the metal on my teeth to be put on correctly, to grant me the perfect smile I had always wanted, and to be set free.

"Well, if you don't, be thankful," she said, snapping the wire back into position now that all of my brackets were in place. "I know they are a blessing, but they will change your life forever and there's just no going back."

I didn't acknowledge her words or pretend to care about her life or her child. I just sat in the chair as electronic knuckles massaged my spine and allowed the pain of my over-stretched cheeks to cover me like a blanket as I closed my eyes and fell into a shallow sleep.

She was there, alive, in my dreams two months later, with a head full of sandy blond hair and eyes the size of thumbprints. She was a hybrid of Boo from *Monster's Inc.,* and Suri Cruise, all blue eyes and dramatic preciousness. Her paisley green jumper, enveloping my face as I nudged my chin into her clothed belly, was the softest cotton I have ever virtually placed against my skin.

I laughed with her as she wrapped her toothless mouth around my chin and sucked on my stubble, grinding her gums into my beard in hopes that milk would emerge. Constance was covered in a blanket of sunlight that seemed to have no source rather; it was a light that simply existed for the sole purpose of illuminating her beauty.

Nothing else happened beyond our happiness, and in toto the dream lasted for what felt like an upbeat, thirty-second commercial for something cheerful. It was the first dream I'd ever had about our child, a dream in which we had a baby and I could hold her in my arms. Holding her, knowing that she was mine, and then waking up empty-handed, wanting nothing more than to have her back, left me hollow and on the brink of tears all day. I craved that same sleep all over again.

She seemed perfect, but she wasn't real and she wasn't ours. Only the real thing, only the life that happens in between lights on and lights out, is worth holding on to, and we continue to wait.

Conclusion

· ·

Even an End Has a Beginning

For those of you craving a happy-ending fix, I'm proud to offer you three: Constance and I are still madly in love, Susan was pronounced cancer-free, and Krista and her family are holding each other closer than ever. Baby remains elusive, but we continue down the line.

During the twelve months we held court with Dr. Leya, Constance and I fell for her rustic charm and no-nonsense care. Even the last time I saw her, when she poked her head through the window separating her offices from the waiting room, I was comforted by her familiar, sincere face and the shoulder-length brown hair that was the pendulum, ticking back and forth, marking time in our disappointing march.

"I hated getting that call yesterday," she said. "I was praying for you guys. I'm just so sorry."

We had officially cycled through two years of periods when none were wanted, and Dr. Leya had been by us for a full lap through four seasons.

Her face was sullen yet determined, and it was in that face and in the countless inappropriate jokes and stories she had shared with us during that time from where we drew the most viable, cost-effective fuel to keep our never-ending drive up the mountain as economical and fun as possible.

Which is why Constance cried on the drive to the Howard Red Line El train stop, and I spent the bulk of my workday at my desk, sullen and moody, after finding out that Dr. Leya does not do IVF. Before we even had the chance to announce our decision to move on, to move ahead to the most promising options, she suggested it was time for Mattstance (our combined name, coined by our friend, Lisa) to go the high-tech route.

"Your count is perfect for IVF, and at your age, Constance, you guys are great candidates," Dr. Leya said. "I'll give you two referrals of places where I send my patients, and you'll just have to check with your insurance to see which one it covers." When Dr. Leya left the room to get us the information for the two offices, and as Constance got dressed, there was very little air or room to breathe. I stared at her ultrasound wand, the wand that had probed and prodded my wife's insides at least seventy times over the last year and couldn't fathom it no longer being a part of my life. The flipbook of STDs, the stack of condoms, the antique scale that hovered in the corner threatening to weigh us upon every visit—this had become our home for all things infertility, and we were getting evicted with zero notice or time to pack up our emotional baggage.

"I guess I never thought about it," Constance said. "That we'd have to leave Dr. Leya. I know it makes sense to go ahead with IVF, and I want to, but I don't know. It seems like we've come to the end of the road and that makes me sad. I just wanted her to fix us. Not somebody else."

I never expected to become invested in our reproductive endocrinologist on a personal level, on a level at which I rooted for a specific doctor to be the hero of this tale. Just like Constance, however, I had envisioned sharing the joy of success with Dr. Leya, of defeating the enemy with her superscientific prowess and crying tears of joy and exhaustion with our wand-wielding savior.

It was more than the inconvenient hassle of switching doctors or telling our story all over again from the start to a new man or woman ready to insert instruments of torture into Constance's vagina. I felt as though I had been reading a comic book and expecting my personal Batman to annihilate evil, but instead of a climactic victory for the good of fertility kind, a demonic ultrasound wand fixed for revenge killed my Batman.

Now more than ever, heading into IVF, I knew that we'd have to be the heroes of our own tale after all.

Our first trip to the Fertility Center of Illinois was nothing short of mechanical. Constance and I were a duo of infertile George Jetsons, thrust from our bed, dragged down the assembly line with our day set in motion without need for exertion or routine. Thoughts or feelings were moot, and had they been expressed, they would have been greeted with the same colloquial disdain given customers abusing the ten-items-or-less lane with a few extra Yoplaits.

It was, in short, perfect. Dr. Koenig, an Australian-born semi-nerd, was all business and could sense the impatience of our glazed-over eyes as he described what it meant to be infertile and what we were going to do to fix it. A tour guide in our own hometown, Dr. Koenig insisted on telling us everything we already knew without once asking if we wanted to be prodded with the reasons behind our failing reproductive organs once again. Our ears didn't perk up until he got to the gravy.

"Every cycle you'll have a fifty to sixty percent chance of conceiving, and at your age you have two choices," he said. "One or two embryos, whatever you're comfortable with, but definitely no more than that."

He never strung words together in the form of a question, so we kept all of the answers to ourselves. We wanted two embryos, and we wanted them straight away. "You guys think about this stuff and decide what you want to do. You don't need to know that for a while."

All he needed was to check our blood to make sure we were

both STD-free before beginning the process. Once Constance got her period, we would be ready to begin a cycle of birth control pills for three weeks headed toward a mid-July embryo transfer.

I never expected to sign my name to a document allowing lab technicians to freeze our embryos in case we want more babies down the line, but I did. I never expected to have my potential child created in a lab without my presence, but it will happen. But the way the clinic is set up, and perhaps by the very nature of IVF, it doesn't really matter what I expected. There's a process, an aggressive regimen of pills, shots, retrievals, sperm washes, growth, and replacement, and very few decisions to be made by the two of us.

It remains a comfort to know the chances are higher and that now we are in an environment noted for getting the job done. What I didn't expect, however, was to be comforted by a more passive decision-making role for the time being. IVF is on its way, and maybe baby, but the journey is no longer totally in our hands. We are "Barren Miss Daisy," and I'm enjoying the view from the backseat, even if we're still driving in that same straight line.

Acknowledgments

· ·

Becoming the man I am today took the hard work of my amazing and patient parents, Marlan and Joy Miller, as well as my older sisters, Angie and April, who always have kept me honest and driven. To my nieces and nephews, Chelsey, Sabastian, Kaela, Ryan, and Aliyah: Your love is a gift. To my in-laws, Richard and Susan Fumea, thank you for giving me the world.

For your astute guidance in life, education, and publishing know-how: Katy Schmitt, Marianne Fons, Dawn Esser, Anne Bartelt, Noel Riley Fitch, Bev Bennett, Mary Connors, Paul Camp, Grace Freedson, Michele Matrisciani, and the entire HCI team.

For your lifetime of friendship: Sarah Zahn, Mary Fons, Orlon Johnson, Lisa Weimai, Krista Thomas, Kyle Barhamand, Cheryl Thoele, Karen Cohen, Blaine McMurry, the entire Content That Works family, Joanna Patterson, Kamila Brodowinska, Jenni Hansen, and Mark Bruscianelli.

For providing the soundtrack to this book's composition: R.E.M., Tori Amos, Patty Griffin, Aimee Mann, Nada Surf, Rilo Kiley, and The National.

Most important . . . to Constance, Marcy, and Cleo—my loving family. And, of course, the inimitable Grandma J.

About the Author

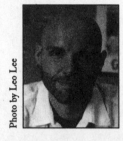

Matthew M. F. Miller is a syndicated blogger, freelance writer, and creative web director for a national newspaper syndicate, where his work has been published in more than 400 newspapers in the United States and Canada, including the *Boston Globe*, *Los Angeles Times*, and *Baltimore Sun*. He holds a master's degree in professional writing from the University of Southern California and was a member of the University of Iowa undergraduate fiction and poetry writers' workshops. Matthew lives in Chicago with his wife, Constance; cat, Cleo; and dog, Marcy.

About the Blog

· ·

Maybebabyblog.com

Maybe Baby was a concept that never once skidded across the radar screen of writer Matthew M. F. Miller. Like any virile twenty-something man, the arrogance of his fertility was a subtle yet strong emotion, mentally catalogued between inane, pride-inducing abilities such as his brisk, chef-like knife skills and a sturdy Norwegian jaw line.

In the spring of 2006, said arrogance led him and his wife, Constance, to commit the single biggest blunder any parents-in-progress can make short of quitting their jobs to pursue full-time uranium mining; they purchased a nursery set for a baby that had yet to be conceived. More than two years later, that three-hundred-dollar nursery set is tucked in a closet alongside a vinyl record collection—a set of useless relics stuffing the gap between the cat litter and an excessive board-game collection.

Maybe Baby began as a humorous syndicated blog to

chronicle their infertility and attempted parenthood and grew rapidly from 700 visits per month to nearly 5,000. Maybe Baby was named a top 5 fatherhood blog by *Parents* magazine in 2007 and is the preeminent male infertility blog on the Internet today, appearing on the websites of more than fifteen newspapers in the United States.

In addition, Mr. Miller's blog has been featured on *Los Angeles Times* website, ePregnancy.com, and in *The New Atlantic* journal. A quarterly Maybe Baby column is syndicated to more than seventy newspapers in the United States and Canada.